Award-winning writer, television broadcaster and author of numerous bestsellers, **Leslie Kenton** is described by the press as 'the guru of health and fitness' and 'the most ori̶ ̶ ̶ce in health'. A shining example of energ̶ ̶ ̶ e is highly respected for her th̶ ̶ ̶ in California, and is th̶ ̶ ̶n. After leaving Stanford ̶ ̶ ̶r early twenties, settling ̶ ̶ s since remained. She h̶ ̶ ̶ ̶ ̶ oy working as a television t̶ ̶ ̶ ̶ ̶ter and teacher on health and for fourte̶ ̶ ̶ was an editor at *Harpers & Queen*.

Leslie's writing on mainstream health is internationally known and has appeared in *Vogue*, the *Sunday Times*, *Cosmopolitan* and the *Daily Mail*. She is the author of many other health books including: *The New Raw Energy* and *Raw Energy Recipes* – co-authored with her daughter Susannah – *The New Biogenic Diet*, *The New Joy of Beauty*, *The New Ageless Ageing*, *Cellulite Revolution*, *10 Day Clean-Up Plan*, *Endless Energy*, *Nature's Child*, *Lean Revolution* and the *10 Day De-Stress Plan*. She turned to fiction with *Ludwig* – her first novel. Former consultant to a medical corporation in the USA and to the Open University's Centre of Continuing Education, Leslie's writing has won several awards including the PPA 'Technical Writer of the Year'. Her work was honoured by her being asked to deliver the McCarrison Lecture at the Royal Society of Medicine. In recent years she has become increasingly concerned not only with the process of enhancing individual health but also with re-establishing bonds with the earth as a part of helping to heal the planet.

THE NEW
ULTRAHEALTH

The positive way to vitality and good looks

LESLIE KENTON

VERMILION
LONDON

1 3 5 7 9 10 8 6 4 2

First published in the United Kingdom in 1995 by
Vermilion
an imprint of Ebury Press
Random House
20 Vauxhall Bridge Road
London SW1V 2SA

Random House Australia (Pty) Limited
20 Alfred Street, Milsons Point, Sydney,
New South Wales 2061, Australia

Random House New Zealand Limited
18 Poland Road, Glenfield,
Auckland 10, New Zealand

Random House South Africa (Pty) Limited
PO Box 337, Bergvlei, South Africa

Random House Canada
1265 Aerowood Drive, Mississauga,
Ontario L4W 1B9, Canada

Random House UK Limited Reg. No. 954009

A CIP catalogue record for this book is available from the
British Library

ISBN: 0 09 178515 4

Photoset by Deltatype Ltd, Ellesmere Port
Printed and bound in Great Britain by Cox & Wyman Ltd,
Reading, Berkshire

Papers used by Ebury Press are natural recyclable products
made from wood grown in sustainable forests.

To Nina Myskow
with admiration and affection

Acknowledgements

This is a book about wellness – that state of being where you feel great and look good – not illness and how to cure it. The information in this book is intended for informational purposes only. None of the suggestions or information is meant in any way to be prescriptive. Any attempt to treat a medical condition should always come under the direction of a competent physician or health practitioner who is familiar with nutritional and exercise therapy – and neither the publisher nor I can accept responsibility for injuries or illness arising out of a failure by a reader to take medical advice. I am only a reporter. I also have a profound interest in helping myself and others to maximize potentials for positive health which includes being able to live at a high level of energy, intelligence and creativity. For all three are expressions of harmony within a living organic system.

Many friends and colleagues have contributed a great deal to make this book possible. It would be impossible to list them all. There are a few to whom I am particularly indebted: Dr Andrew Strigner, Dr Gordon Latto, Dr Barbara Latto, Dr Dagmar Liechti von Brasch, Dr John Kane, Dr Phillip Kilsby, Dr Siegmund Schmidt, Graham Jones, Tony Wall, Vera Diamond, Dr Malcolm Curruthers and my daughter Susannah, whose energy, cheerfulness (except at 6am) and hard work is an inspiration to me in my own search for ultrahealth.

Leslie Kenton
Pembrokeshire 1995

Contents

Six: The Ultra Face

Seven: The Body Beautiful

Eight: Get It Together

PART ONE

ULTRAHEALTH VS 20TH CENTURY LIFE

1
The Master Game

DID YOU EVER wonder what it was like to feel great most of the time? To awaken in the mornings looking forward to each day? To work hard but have plenty of energy to spare at the end of the day for play? To look terrific and to feel good about yourself and your life? To know you have everything you need to meet whatever challenge you may face? Sounds like a utopian dream? It's not. It is something within your grasp – something called ultrahealth.

What is Ultrahealth?
It is not the same thing as preventative medicine nor is it medical self-care, or holistic medicine. Preventative medicine is mainly concerned with avoiding illness, holistic health is primarily aimed at treatment – although the treatment of the whole person rather than specific symptoms. Medical self-care aims to make a person able to diagnose and take care of his or her own minor medical problems. Although ultrahealth can share in some of the benefits of all three, in a strong sense it is still very different and goes far beyond them. For ultrahealth does not focus primarily on disease or its prevention. Instead, its major thrust is a deliberate choice on the part of the person practising it to live at the peaks – to explore the *heights* – of wellbeing: physically, emotionally and in the full use of his or her creative potentials. In fact the choice for living at the peaks is one which an increasing number of people in developed countries are making. This is evident in our growing desire for high-level fitness, for longer and more active lives, for improving and preserving our good looks and for consistent higher energy levels. Where in 1970 an ambitious man or woman might have wanted more recognition,

money and possessions, in the Nineties these are not enough. Instead he or she wants to make the most of their own potentials in every possible way. Ultrahealth aims at the enjoyable and often amusing search for peaks of whole-person functioning. As such it is its own goal and its own reward. And the process of moving towards it can be as much fun as the achievements of its ends.

Playing the Game

Seeking ultrahealth is a kind of game. And like any game it has its players, its obstacles, its rules, its rewards, its penalties, and a goal. The *Shorter Oxford Dictionary* defines game as 'amusement, fun, sport . . . a diversion of the nature of a contest played according to the rules and decided by superior skill, strength, or good fortune'. The ultrahealth game is just like that. In many ways it is probably the most rewarding bit of amusement you can indulge in – a real 'master game'. This is not only because playing to win can keep you looking and feeling vital and young longer after the 'losers' have been left by the wayside, but because, like all good games, the play itself can be so interesting and so challenging. It can also demand considerable skill. Some people will find ultrahealth easy – they seem to have a natural flair for the challenge or without realizing it they already know lots of the rules and manoeuvres. Others will have to work harder at it. But it is often those who have to work the hardest that seem to get the greatest satisfaction from play and who make the most dramatic improvements in the long run.

The Tools for Play

What are they? First, they're *information* about how various techniques, practices and attitudes – such as dietary factors, relaxation skills, exercise, political responsibility and special treats and treatments – can contribute to optimal wellness. What are you playing against? Time. Perhaps your genes too. Some people will find their genetic inheritance an asset to the play, others will have to compensate for what they didn't get at birth with more effort and more awareness of how to make the best possible use of what they have been given. One of the major obstacles to ultrahealth in the Nineties is the kind of environmental pollution we are all exposed to. To counter it you not only need to increase your awareness of its dangers and use counter agents – such as the natural substances and anti-oxidant nutrients – which can help defeat its negative effect on your body. You may also need to take social and political action to ensure that your water, air and food supplies are not further denatured by environmental toxins and radiation.

Another major obstacle to the goals of ultrahealth is indifference; the tendency we all have to go along with cultural and social norms. Why not live on fast foods and chocolate bars since so many do? It is easier than seeking out a fresh crisp salad. Why not indeed? The ultrahealth player will tell you very clearly – because such a way of eating is part of a lifestyle that does not help you reach your goal of high-level wellness and peak functioning, mentally and emotionally. As such it is better off discarded.

A Quick Guide to Playing the Ultrahealth Game

- **The Goal**: High-level health
- **What are you playing against?**
  Time
  Your genetic inheritance
  Environmental pollution
  Cultural norms
  Indifference
  Ignorance
  Wrong notions about health
- **What are the tools for play?**
  Information
  Understanding the rules
  Diet
  Exercise
  Special treats and treatments
  Relaxation techniques
  Political responsibility

Doing Battle With False Notions

And who are your opponents in the game? There are many. For instance, people who are content to allow time to take its course or those who assume that as the years pass your body and your good looks inevitably deteriorate and that chronic illness is a natural part of old age. False notions about health can also be major opponents:

the idea that responsibility for your health rests not with yourself but with your doctor or your mother or the state. The notion that ultrahealth demands too many sacrifices and is not rewarding enough – might take too much time for too little fun – is another fierce opponent. But the *worst* opponent of all is a lack of belief in your ability to play the game. Lots of people just don't believe that ultrahealth is possible for them. 'We are', they say, 'too old', 'too fat', 'too lazy', 'too busy'. In fact just the opposite is probably true. Learn to play the game, create an ultrahealth way of life for yourself and all those 'toos' will vanish leaving you much more time and energy than you had before. Ultrahealth is a game you need no previous experience to play. You begin wherever you are right now and you gradually build your knowledge of the game's rules and your own skills until in time you can far surpass someone who seemed infinitely better endowed than you at the beginning. For human life is never static – either you are getting better or you are getting worse. And as with any game, how fast you progress, and how many rewards you get from playing, depend to a large extent on how much fun you find it and how hard you are willing to play.

Playing the ultrahealth game also keeps health in perspective. For being healthy, like being alive, should be challenging, exciting and fun. Don't let yourself become self-righteous or self-obsessed, and the fun will go on and on.

Let's Define the Field of Play

Most people think of health as a state in which you are not ill, you are free of pain and you show no signs or symptoms of the development of disease. In other words, health is really a state characterized by the absence of something – namely sickness. So long as this is true they figure all things are well (touch wood) and they go about their business until at some later date (they figure), if they are not lucky, they may inadvertently be struck down. This rather tenuous state called 'health' will suddenly turn into its opposite – *'illness'*.

Thinking of health in this way can be very limiting: the best you can hope for is 'non-sickness'. Ultrahealth players take a different point of view. They work from larger models. They not only believe that by taking control of their own way of living they can avoid becoming ill, they know that the high-level wellness they are aiming for has positive attributes far beyond the absence of disease. They see that it encompasses high levels of fitness, good looks and wellbeing and takes in the peaks as well as the depths. But it is primarily the peaks they are interested in. Not content with being 'un-sick', they want high levels of energy – to be able to work and play hard, and to have the kind of mental clarity that makes possible the full use of their creative potentials. Their paradigms of reality include a notion which to many people seems quite foreign: that *you* are the prime cause of what happens to your health and your life, not blind fate. Without such a commitment to autonomy no player in the ultrahealth game is likely to become a winner. With such a commitment, the sky is virtually the limit. There is no reason why you should not be fit at 90, look twenty years younger than your peers at 70 and feel terrific. It is all a matter of developing the right game and playing with the knowledge and determination of a pro.

The Six Facets of Ultrahealth

The ultrahealth lifestyle has six major facets to it: nutritional action, physical fitness, stress management, self-responsibility, age control and environmental awareness. The chapters which follow deal with different aspects of these major dimensions. They also offer advice on how to 'get-it-all-together' to make all six work for you. Their advice is in no sense meant to replace proper medical care if you are ill. What it can do is provide you with some of the tools to help you develop your own style of play in the ultrahealth game and to play it well. I hope that the following chapters will help give you a feel for just how much fun it can be.

Ultrahealth as a Key to Freedom

This morning I went for a run, as I often do, along the cliffs in Pembrokeshire where we live. After running for about three miles I suddenly had an impulse to plunge into the sea and swim back. It was something that I had never done before. But the sun was warm and the sea calmer than usual so I did – running shoes and all. An hour later I found myself back on our home beach – fingers tingling with the cold and legs a little wobbly, trying to make that transition from the world of water which I'd been moving through to the thinner air-medium of land. But I felt great. And I loved the feeling of freedom that it brought me – a strong sense of my own physical limits and a knowledge that they are considerably broader than they were ten years ago before I myself became so involved in the ultrahealth game. But why did I do it? To prove I could? Not really. I had few doubts on that account. To make myself fitter and stronger? I had no such notions in my head. I did it for the sheer pleasure of it. It was the same impulse that makes children climb trees. Not to get to the top but just for fun.

The Six Facets of Ultrahealth

- Self-responsibility
- Nutritional action
- Physical fitness
- Age control
- Stress management
- Environmental awareness

Why Play the Ultrahealth Game?

The serious answer goes something like this: so you will feel better, look younger, have more energy and probably even live longer. And indeed all those things are true. But once you get involved in the play you realize that something much more exciting is happening than trying to reach these goals. You are having fun. Grasp even a little of that sense and you are half way to your goal already. Make that kind of fun a part of your life and the rules of the ultrahealth game, which at the beginning may have had to be tediously learnt one by one, become second nature. Meanwhile, just playing the game starts to be something so rich and so delightful that you can forget all about goals. Then it's the play itself that matters.

2
Step One: Getting Ready for Play

ONE OF THE first steps in learning the ultrahealth game is sorting out how it relates to the orthodox medical system, defining the capabilities of doctors, drugs, clinics and hospitals and delineating what role they should play in your life. The notion that all modern medicine should be dismissed in favour of some radical 'alternative therapy' is rather like throwing out the baby with the bath water. Used well, the medical system plays an important part in achieving optimal health. But problems arise when expectations exceed the limits of medical capabilities.

Making the Medical System Work *For* You, Not *Against* You
The medical system which we in the west have inherited focuses almost entirely on pathology. It functions within the realm of the unwell. And, despite some rather brave attempts in very recent years to incorporate such things as dietary warnings against eating too much fat and sugar and too little fibre, in a bid to reduce deaths from coronary heart disease and cancer, modern medicine does little to foster the development of healthy lifestyles in its patients. What it *is* good at – indeed better than any medical system in the history of the world – is the diagnosis of pathology. It is also extremely efficient when it comes to dramatic interventions such as coronary bypass operations designed to save lives, and it has developed sophisticated biomedical technology involving such things as kidney dialysis and prosthetic joints. The pathological orientation of our medical-scientific system has also made possible the control of widespread infectious diseases through vaccination, the development of antibiotic drugs and improved public hygiene.

Many of the techniques of modern medicine can be profoundly reassuring to a sick patient who needs explanations and help in his predicament. It is in these capacities that one needs to make use of such a medical system. Then it is capable of serving you well. The difficulty comes when your expectations of it do not coincide with what it has to offer. That's why it is just as important to understand what it *can't* do as what it *can*.

The areas of illness in which our medical system has still made little progress are those which have come to be known as 'the diseases of civilization' – degenerative diseases such as cardio-vascular disease, cancer, arthritis and respiratory ailments, including emphysema and bronchitis as well as depressive mental states – all of which have increased dramatically in the last half century. Advances in the treatment and prevention of these illnesses have been very slow indeed, in some cases almost negligible, because the causes of these illnesses lie beyond the realms that our medical system can significantly influence: in your genetic disposition, in environmental contamination and, most important of all, in the way you live. This includes how you eat, rest, think, exercise, and generally look after yourself. In order to prevent such illnesses all the self-neglecting or self-destructive elements of your lifestyle need to change. And, while certain diagnostic tests may be useful in determining which areas need changing, our sophisticated bio-medical technology with all its drugs and diagnostic tools offers little or no help in making such changes. For our medical system does not even concern itself with measuring or studying optimal physical and mental states in the human being. Indeed it knows very little about them.

Don't Confuse Positive Health with Good Medical Care

Good medical care is essential in life-threatening situations but it does not lead to *positive* health – a state of optimal functioning which keeps you free from degenerative illness and premature ageing. Only *you* can be responsible for that. Also you only can decide exactly what kind of intervention from the medical system is appropriate. That is why it is important that each of us be as well-informed as possible about what alternatives are available before consenting to any form of medical treatment. It is also why second opinions of medical experts are so valuable in deciding for or against medical interventions such as surgery, or the use of drugs which can have powerful side-effects. The medical system is only as good as the use to which you put it. Under-used, it can cause loss of life. Over-used, used wrongly or without awareness of consequences, it can result in *iatrogenic* diseases, side-effects and the superficial treatment of symptoms while the underlying condition only worsens.

Two other things are important to remember as well. First, most non-serious illnesses are self-limiting. They need no medical intervention for cure. Allowed to run its course, provided you rest a little and go easy on rich foods, a cold or 'flu will come to an end and leave you feeling slightly weaker perhaps, but often lighter and better than you did before it arrived. To interfere too much with that course can create more health problems than it will solve. Second, symptoms such as headaches, back pains, fever, and the like probably *mean* something. They are a way that your body has of telling you that something is wrong. Listen to them as if they were messages from your 'control centre'. Gradually you will develop a kind of awareness of your own body and its needs which will eventually make many of the 'rules' for ultrahealth seem pedantic. After all, who needs to read the rules when you already know a game well? With practice at playing they become second nature. Then, what Jung called 'intuition' takes over. You tend to do the right thing automatically.

What the Medical System Can and Can't Do

It Can

- Diagnose a wide range of problems
- Treat symptoms
- Tend to injuries – sprains, broken bones etc.
- Replace secretions of worn-out glands
- Supply artificial aids for hearing and sight and replace limbs, joints etc.
- Arrest some pathological states
- Save lives (at least for short periods of time) e.g. kidney dialysis, surgical heart bypass operations

It Can't

- Successfully cure many 'diseases of civilization' including cancer, cardiovascular diseases, emphysema etc.
- Provide preventative medical care
- Cure many psychological illnesses such as depression
- PROMOTE HIGH-LEVEL WELLNESS OR ULTRAHEALTH

Caution: Unconscious Assumptions May Damage Your Health

Another 'first step' in the ultrahealth game is examining just what kind of unconscious assumptions, social expectations, belief systems and values are influencing you in your choice of the way you live your life right now. These values or 'norms' are things which we rarely think about, although the effects they have on our life and health can be pervasive. There are all sorts of unspoken cultural values implicit in our society which, for better or for worse (usually for worse), exert a profound influence on our health. It is important to know what they are. It can be extremely difficult to change a lifestyle which is oriented to 'worseness' into one directed towards 'wellness' unless you gradually alter your response to the most common life-eroding cultural values. For instance, have you ever noticed that in almost every Hollywood film about the beautiful people the first thing any of them do on entering a room is fix a drink? Advertisements are full of similar implications – that drinking a certain kind of rum or vermouth will bring you a taste of the exciting jet-set life, while cigarette smoking is still toted in some circles as the ultimate in urbane sophistication. And even if you don't smoke yourself you are subjected to smoke pollution in restaurants, dinner parties and perhaps in your own home because in some countries smoking, like alcohol, is still an important part of the values implicit in our culture. The food ads you and your children see are usually full of junk-food – crunchy breakfast cereals dripping with refined sugar, slimming products, 'adult' ice creams, supposedly energy-giving chocolate bars and highly-processed, ready-in-a-minute dinners which are very low in nutritional value. From practically every angle advertisers are seducing us with implicit cultural values that can do damage to your looks and are destructive to high-level health.

Wellness Can Be a Social Threat

And just in case you think you are not influenced by these values, try going to a party and drinking nothing but mineral water. You're likely to arouse a great deal of irritation from friends and acquaintances. People can feel threatened by those who go against their cultural values. After all, 'Who do they think they are? Some kind of superior person? I've been drinking three glasses of whisky every day for the past 20 years and just look at me, I am the picture of health.' Other implicit cultural values which are health-eroding include the notion that physical exercise is something 'down-market', that a sedentary lifestyle has particular charm (especially for women whose femininity can be threatened by perspiration), that a 'good meal' consists of rich fatty foods, not fresh light salads and fruits, that it is normal to wake up in the morning feeling lousy until you've had your cup of coffee, that work is something to be avoided, that two eggs and sausage constitute a 'healthy breakfast', that it is normal to live and work in a polluted atmosphere, that to be an adult means to accept the responsibility of a 'hard' life, and that to grow older means inevitable illness. 'I mean, doesn't everybody get ill as they get older?'

Values for Wellness or Worseness?

Such unconscious assumptions are powerful forces for promoting low-level health. Start to change your lifestyle by beginning to play the ultrahealth game and you'll be amazed what a pull they exert on you even if you don't consciously agree with any one of them. So often people with good intentions for improving their health and the quality of their life come a cropper because of the immense social pressures those around them exert through such implicit values. Then they accuse themselves of being weak-willed and tend to give up their intentions or to fall back into their old life-destroying ways of being. In truth they have been secretly overwhelmed by the non-supportive environment in which they live. It is not easy to resist the temptation to maintain the status quo. Going along with things is the path of least resistance. It is because of these implicit health-destroying values that you can have so much trouble when you start on a programme which will do you good in staying on it. The pull of mediocrity is a potent force for 'worseness'.

'Wellness' Values

- The focus of a main meal should be fresh vegetables, whole-grains and pulses plus a large mixed salad, preferably containing sprouted seeds, pulses, grains
- It is normal to wake up happy and energetic and feel good about your life and work
- It is normal not to be ill and to grow old without becoming ill or crippled
- It is normal to be slim and to look your best most of the time

'Worseness' Values

- A good dinner is *hot* and contains lots of protein, such as beef or pork, plus a few boiled vegetables
- It is normal to be depressed and tired and to look forward only to weekends, holidays and promotions
- It is normal to have 'flu or a cold at least four times a year and to expect a serious illness or disease after the age of 50 or so
- It is normal to look tired, run down or out of shape and only to look really good after a two-week holiday break

Altering 'Norms'

How then does one make changes for ultrahealth? By becoming some kind of hero or martyr? There are few of either. Most people who have a desire to play the ultrahealth game have no inclination towards either role. The alternative is to become aware of just what kind of underlying assumptions and social 'norms' may be influencing you away from high-level health. This awareness itself makes them lose a lot of their power. It also helps to remember that these values, no matter how long they have been operative, are in no sense *permanent*. Think back fifteen years ago when it was absolutely not acceptable for a woman to be seen running on the roads in a track suit and how now track suits and training shoes, the symbols of physical activity, have become the 'in' mode of trendy casual dress. Be aware of the kind of assumptions you have about health too. Are they, like most people's, based on the notion that to be healthy is not to be ill or do they go beyond that? Open yourself to new ideas. Seek out others with whom you share some of the newer health-promoting values – for instance drinking mineral water with a twist of lime instead of gin and tonic at Sunday drinks parties, exercising several times a week at a gym or running in the park daily. Have you ever noticed how much easier it is to follow health-promoting habits when you are with other people who do? Explore low-fat cooking as a hobby instead of turning out rich old-fashioned French dishes at dinner parties.

You don't need to be a hero to play the ultrahealth game. But you do need to be aware of cultural norms and implicit assumptions which pressure you into mediocrity and you need quietly but firmly to resist them. If you're clever you can turn your newer, more health-promoting habits into something others will actually copy, provided you drink the mineral water with flair, and pursue your lifestyle with individual enthusiasm and fun. This is the perfect time to do it. Never in the history of the western world has there been so much interest in health. The ultrahealth game is one a lot of people will be trying to play in ten years' time. Start now and you can be a trend setter.

What's Ultrahealth Like?

All of us know a lot about illness even if we have never been seriously ill. We're bombarded with information from the media about the suffering of cancer victims, the 'warning signs' of diabetes or arthritis or coronary heart disease and filled full of information about all the stuff we have to avoid (like too much cholesterol, too many eggs, too much alcohol and so forth). But we are almost never told what it is like to be optimally well. Indeed high-level wellness is a state which, unlike disease, has been little studied. The scientific community has chosen to ignore defining it altogether. Only a few humanistic and transpersonal psychologists such as Abraham Maslow, Roberto Assiogioli and Carl Rogers have attempted to delineate its characteristics. So we are in a position of having our consciousness filled with a lot of stuff about illness but virtually devoid of any images of what it means to be truly well. If you are going to play the ultrahealth game, this needs to change. You need to start thinking about wellness and imagining what optimal health will be like for you. You need to introduce yourself to positive realms of possibility which gradually, through using the ultrahealth tools, can become reality for you. In other words, before you can set off for your goal of high-level wellness you've got to have a pretty good idea of how it's going to be for you when you arrive. The better your appreciation of this goal is, the easier that ultrahealth game becomes. Let's look at a few *new* images which, instead of working against you as so many of our negative cultural assumptions do, can work for you.

- *Feeling good means energy to spare.* Not having to think about whether or not you can cope. Not having to forgo some pleasant event because you are likely to be too tired after work to want to go out again.

- *Mornings are good times, not bad.* Remember what it's like to be a child? To wake up in the morning with a feeling of anticipation about the day ahead? To wonder just how many good new things it will bring? That is not some half-made state reserved for kids and fools, these are some of the things you feel when you are optimally healthy.

- *Ultrahealth means high-level fitness.* Stamina is built into the ultrahealth lifestyle. Your body is firm and strong and in good shape. You will face exercise not as a chore but with enjoyment, taking pleasure in the feel of your body and the way it moves as you want it to.

- *Freedom from addictions* is also part of high-level wellness. You will be in control of your life and what you do with it, not at the mercy of compulsive eating, alcohol drinking and cigarette smoking.

- *High self-esteem* is inherent in ultrahealth. When people feel well, fit and in control, their sense of self improves.

- *Truly healthy people have a balanced lifestyle* where everything seems to fit. They are neither fanatical nor rigid and tolerate those whose values differ from theirs.

- *A sense of purpose and meaning is part of ultrahealth.* Nihilism and indifference very much belong not to wellness but to worseness – that 'other world' – of addiction, poor health habits and lowered self-esteem. Feeling well brings a positive sense of meaning to your outlook on life.

- *Ultrahealth means ultra good looks as well.* You know what it is like to return from a relaxing holiday or a health farm where you've just lost 10 pounds and everybody you meet seems to tell you how great you look? That is how optimally healthy people look most of the time. They age more slowly than their friends who are worseness- rather than wellness-oriented. Their skin is clearer and their eyes brighter. Ultrahealth is worth more than the most expensive and elaborate face lifts if you care about how you look.

Where Do You Belong on the Wellness to Worseness Scale?
Before you begin learning the ultrahealth skills it is useful to discover just exactly where you stand now. The following quiz will give you some idea how near or far you are from reaching ultrahealth goals and give you some points of comparison for you to judge your values and beliefs against. The quiz, which should be done light-heartedly despite its serious purposes, is divided into 6 sections each containing questions on one of the ultrahealth facets. Read through the questions and then turn to pages 25–6 to find out how you scored.

QUIZ

Nutritional action
1. When you buy a product at the supermarket and you find a list of contents including: dextrose, glucose syrup, edible starch, permitted flavouring, artificial colouring, preservatives . . . do you:
a) Toss the food into your shopping trolley without hesitation?
b) Pause thoughtfully over 'edible' and 'permitted' and then decide it must be safe otherwise the government wouldn't allow it?
c) Quickly replace it on the shelf next to the detergents and look for a *real* food?

2. How do you restrict your intake of refined sugar?
a) I don't – in any case, I don't need to because I'm not fat.
b) I take saccharine or *just a little* sugar in my tea and coffee and *try* to avoid chocolate and sweets.
c) I avoid all foods that contain refined sugar and substitute honey or unrefined sugar in recipes and drinks.

3. What is your attitude to vitamin and mineral supplements?

a) They are for health freaks – I don't need them.

b) I eat a well-balanced diet so I don't have to take any.

c) I see them as a useful option for finely tuning a body to achieve peak performance.

4. Do you include plenty of roughage in your diet?

a) Isn't that something people eat to lose weight?

b) Yes, I sprinkle bran on my breakfast cereal and sometimes stir it into a glass of milk or juice . . . then I can eat white bread and cakes and not worry about getting enough fibre.

c) I include lots of fresh raw vegetables and fruits in my diet for fibre. Bran? Who needs it!

5. Do you eat yourself, give your children and infants (or allow them to have): commercial baby food, convenience frozen foods, soft drinks, sweets, biscuits, cakes etc.?

a) Yes.

b) Some of these.

c) None of these.

6. What is your idea of a well-balanced diet?

a) Lots of protein – meat, eggs, milk, cheese and a hearty cooked breakfast to start the day.

b) Lots of protein, cooked veggies, bran and not too much sugar.

c) Comparatively little protein and fat, lots of raw vegetables, whole grains, and fresh fruits.

7. Standing at a kiosk you feel a little hungry and decide to have a quick snack. Do you:

a) Reach for a glucose-enriched chocolate bar to give you energy?

b) Choose a ham sandwich even though the bread looks a little stale – at least it will fill you up?

c) Pick a crunchy apple to sustain you until your next meal without interfering with your digestion?

8. What are the most important considerations when you choose a meal?

a) Something to leave you feeling full – a hamburger with chips, followed by a chocolate sundae and coffee, works wonders.

b) Something really tasty – you'll overlook the added sugar, monosodium glutamate, saturated fats etc. as long as it tastes really good.

c) Taste, sight and smell of the food are important, of course, but you also consider how the meal will leave you feeling afterwards – light, refreshed and energized, or tired and irritable and suffering from indigestion.

Stress Management

9. What is your response to the fact that certain yogis have the capacity to alter so-called 'involuntary' body functions such as blood pressure, heart-rate, glandular secretions, body temperature etc.?
a) What a load of rubbish!
b) They probably can, although it does sound a little bizarre – not something a 'normal' person could do.
c) Such things are indeed possible and can be learnt by anyone. I know they are also used in biofeedback methods for stress control. Maybe they could be useful for me.

10. How do you deal with a headache?
a) Take an aspirin, of course – it will relieve the pain in minutes.
b) Take an aspirin – it can't do any harm because everybody takes aspirins – and headaches really are a nuisance.
c) Realize that there is a *reason* for having a headache, that it is a manifestation of tension or some kind of biochemical imbalance and try to discover why you have it. Then lie down in a quiet dark room for ten minutes with a cool cloth across your forehead and eyes, or have someone gently massage the back of your neck to relieve the muscle tension and lessen the pain.

11. You find yourself at 'boiling point', unable to cope with the stress of a situation – perhaps a confrontation with an irritating relative or a business partner. Do you:
a) Have a drink of scotch, swallow a tranquillizer, smoke several cigarettes and mutter curses under your breath?
b) Eat your way through a packet of biscuits, then beat up a pillow?
c) Go for a walk or find a room where you can be alone and do some deep breathing exercises. Then look at the situation objectively from a distance and decide on the best solution?

12. How often do you feel depressed?
a) I am frequently depressed, often without knowing why – I just feel 'down'.
b) I suffer occasional bad bouts of depression – usually there is a reason for them, but when I get depressed there is really nothing I can do to feel better except wait miserably for the depression to lift.
c) Rarely, and if I do I never lose sight of feeling happy. I can usually pull myself out of it very quickly.

13. How do you cope with depression?
a) Take the pills the doctor has prescribed.
b) Try to get by and take my mind off the problem.
c) Consider why I am depressed and, if the depression might be biochemically linked, detoxify my system or my head to get rid of the pressures that are keeping me from feeling good. Realize what a waste of time feeling depressed is and take action to alleviate the feeling – maybe listen to a beautiful piece of music or go to see a fun film.

14. Do you have trouble sleeping?
a) Usually.
b) Sometimes.
c) Almost never.

15. What do you do when you can't sleep?
a) Have a drink or two and stay up until I can't keep my eyes open any longer, or take a sleeping pill and lie in bed worrying about not falling asleep.
b) Read a boring book for hours, continually turning off and on the light when I realize that I am *still* not sleepy.
c) Drink a cup of warm herb tea and then go to bed. Do a relaxation exercise for ten minutes until my whole body feels relaxed and at peace. And then if I don't sleep it really doesn't matter.

Physical fitness
16. What function do you think exercise serves?
a) It's only useful if you want to lose weight or get bulging biceps – really for how you look.
b) It is important to keep fit so that you reduce the risk of coronary heart disease and to keep slim.

c) Exercise not only keeps your body looking good, but it is important in stimulating all of your bodily functions. It can clear your head as well as improve your digestion and glandular system.

17. What is your attitude towards exercise?
a) I avoid it like the plague. It's uncomfortable and just not my kind of thing.
b) I endure it up to a point, but find it a chore and very boring.
c) I really enjoy it. I not only like the exercise itself, I also value the great way it leaves me feeling. In fact, if I don't get enough exercise I don't feel myself.

18. Do you make a conscious effort to get enough exercise each week?
a) No, I don't think it's that important to worry about. I occasionally walk to work but I just don't have time for exercise – I never was any good at sports at school.
b) I try to play squash or tennis once a week and sometimes go to an evening fitness class, but I really don't have the time or energy to do something every day.
c) I make regular exercise part of my everyday life. I find that it uplifts me and leaves me with the strength and energy to face the demands of the day. I usually do at least 30 minutes of aerobic exercise each day as well as limbering and stretching.

19. Do you feel good about your body?
a) No, but what can I do. I was born this way.
b) Not really, but I try to keep in shape.
c) I feel good about the way I look and find that I feel better and better about myself and my life all the time.

Self-Responsibility
20. How heavily do you rely on the medical system?
a) I do whatever my doctor tells me – he knows best.
b) I sometimes question a prescription I have been given, but am always satisfied that it is what is best for me.
c) I find I need to rely very little on my doctor and tend only to see him when there is an emergency. Even then I am careful to ask exactly what I am being given. Usually I will refuse drugs or antibiotics and look for a natural alternative.

21. In the last couple of months have you read a book on health, natural foods, exercise, meditation etc.?
a) No, I'm not really interested in those kind of books.
b) I've flicked through a couple in bookshops.
c) Yes, I take an interest in reading books related to achieving and maintaining optimum health.

22. Do you have a fundamental knowledge of your physiology – how your food is digested, your breathing mechanism, hormonal system, liver functions, muscles, etc.?
a) I have no idea what goes on inside me except that I have two kidneys and a liver . . . or is it one kidney and two livers?
b) I know the basic lay-out of my body organs, but I'm not sure what most of them do or how they work.
c) I understand fairly well the fundamental body processes and am sensitive to problems in specific areas, for example, I can recognize when my adrenal glands have been temporarily 'exhausted' or my nervous system feels jangled and then take action to restore the balance.

23. You are told that you have a serious tumour which could be cancerous. Do you:
a) Put yourself entirely in the hands of your doctor and accept surgery or chemotherapy as inevitable.
b) Worry about the side-effects of medical treatment, but basically leave things to the 'professionals'.
c) Seek a second opinion. Ask yourself if there are workable complements or alternatives to surgery and drugs – and look for more holistic ways of strengthening your body's immune system so that it can fight the growth itself.

24. You are told that you have an allergy to gluten in wheat flour. You arrive at a dinner party and find that the main course is breaded fish. Do you:
a) Eat the fish anyway – you don't really care about allergies.
b) Decide you can't be rude or difficult and eat the fish, even though you later regret your decision.
c) Politely refuse the fish, explaining your problem. You know that it is important to put your health before social niceties.

25. Do you ever write a journal about how you feel or the things you think?
a) Never – there's no point.
b) I've tried once or twice, but couldn't keep it up.
c) I often record my ideas, thoughts and feelings. By writing a journal I find myself more in touch with my beliefs and goals and can organize my life more effectively.

26. What is your self-image like and how is it affected by those around you?
a) I rarely feel good about myself unless someone pays me a compliment.
b) I feel OK about myself, but I need to rely on other people to boost my self-confidence when I feel down.
c) I feel good about myself most of the time without anyone telling me I look good or do things well.

27. When was the last time you laughed a deep belly laugh?
a) I can't remember.
b) I often laugh, but very seldom let myself go completely (unless I've been drinking).
c) I often find myself smiling for no reason, just because I feel happy, and laugh aloud over the simplest things.

Age control
28. What is your attitude to ageing?
a) It happens to us all eventually – there's nothing much we can do about it.
b) I don't want to get old and will try to postpone the inevitable for as long as possible.
c) I don't see wrinkles, grey hair, disease, chronic illness and crippling as inevitable occurrences in the process of getting older. With knowledge and the right lifestyle ageing can be a healthy process of maturation rather than one of decaying degeneration.

29. Looking in the mirror you find that you have several grey hairs. Do you:
a) Tear them out frantically?
b) Rush out and buy some hair colour?

c) Look at dietary supplements such as PABA which may reduce the rate of hair discolouration or consider that you may look better if you allow your hair to grey?

30. Looking in the mirror you realize that the wrinkles of old age are already creeping across your face. Do you:
a) Say 'Too bad' and pack on the makeup or make a resolution to stay out of bright light when photographs are taken.
b) Decide to save up for plastic surgery when things get really bad.
c) Wonder if through regular exercise, the ultrahealth diet and perhaps the use of anti-oxidant nutrients you can actually fade lines and have your skin looking years younger, then take steps to find out how.

Environmental awareness

31. Are you aware of the damage which the sun's ultraviolet rays can do to you?
a) I think being in the sun is good for you – it makes you look healthy.
b) I sunbathe when I get the chance or use a sun bed. I sometimes use a sun tan lotion to speed up my tan.
c) I am careful to use a sun screen on my face whenever I am in strong sun light and always avoid getting burnt. I am aware of the dangers of skin cancer and rapid ageing caused by exposure to UV rays.

32. Are you aware of water pollution and do you drink tap water?
a) I drink tap water because it has chlorine which kills all the bacteria, so it is perfectly safe.
b) I don't think there is any harm in drinking tap water – everyone does.
c) I avoid drinking tap water because of the hazardous compounds that are formed from certain industrial pollutants which most water purification systems don't remove. Also because of compounds such as chlorine and fluorine that are added to it. I use bottled spring water or filter my own.

33. You are offered a job in an ideal situation with good pay and excellent promotion possibilities. The one drawback is that you have to come in contact with substances which have been proven to be carcinogenic. Do you:

a) Accept the job – I don't worry about pollution.
b) Accept the job – at least for a few years. If I get ill I can always change then.
c) Refuse the job on principle – my health comes before an enticing salary.

34. You read on the front page of your newspaper that the wastes from a local factory are contaminating the air with lead and that this is leading to mental illness in children from nearby schools. Do you:
a) Turn the page?
b) Knowing that vitamin C and kelp are good for protecting against air pollution, make sure you and your family take plenty?
c) Write to your local MP and try to initiate action against the pollution as well?

35. How do you view this quiz?
a) A novel way of killing time.
b) A way of judging how healthy I am.
c) A way of making me more aware of different health hazards and health boosters, the knowledge of which will help me improve my wellness lifestyle.

How did you score?
a) scores 0
b) scores 5
c) scores 10
Add up your score and find which of the three score ranges you fall under.

If you scored between 185 and 360 Congratulations! You have an excellent approach to overall health and have probably reached the stage where you realize just how fun the ultrahealth game can be to play. You can now go on to discover new and exciting ways of achieving your potential in the six dimensions of ultrahealth. You might check to see which particular area you were weak in (if any) and then concentrate particularly on the chapters concerned with it.

If you scored 95–180, depending on how high your score fell in this range, you probably have some sense of the importance of caring for your body and a moderate interest in several of the health fields. You are likely to be someone who vacillates between feeling ill to feeling sort of well to feeling just a little unwell, never quite believing that you are in control of your own health. You are moderately interested in your wellbeing, but have not yet begun to explore the fascinating realm of ultrahealth, practically or even, really, in theory.

If you scored between 0–90 you have quite a way to go up the ultrahealth 'ladder' before you can reach the rewards or bonuses of the game – but do not despair. Very often the motivation to play the ultrahealth game comes out of illness or being fed up with continually being plagued by fatigue and lacking energy. Most of the ultrahealth experts have been helped to reach their goals having experienced the undesirable state of 'underhealth' and rejecting it.

The purpose of this quiz is not to praise the high scorers while scolding the low scorers – the scoring parameters are very rough and not especially important. What matters is that you have some example of the ultrahealth way of life to compare your own lifestyle to and that the questions arouse your curiosity about issues in the six different health fields. You will be able to look back on your score after a few weeks and see just how much you have learnt and how much closer you have come to achieving the ultrahealth goals.

3
Staying Healthy in an Unhealthy World

IT IS NOT only mental phenomena – underlying assumptions and social habit patterns – which create obstacles for someone wanting to pursue an ultrahealth lifestyle. The basic fabric of human existence is now, in simple physical and chemical ways, threatened by many forms of environmental pollution which can have a powerful impact on lowering wellness. It is little wonder that some people suffer from the ultimate twentieth-century paranoia, believing that 'everything is out to get you'. In quite a real sense they are probably right. And while no great boost for wellness can come from spending your time dwelling on how dangerous it all is, a realistic awareness of negative environmental influences, rather than the 'stick-your-head-in-the-ground-like-an-ostrich' response, characteristic of many governments and otherwise intelligent, informed people, can not only help change some of the threats into benefits, it can help you personally counteract them. You should know for instance that environmental pollutants from our foods, water and air as well as many of our daily habits – cigarette smoking to coffee drinking and regular cocktails – are major 'agers' as well as powerful agents that undermine high-level wellness. They do this in part because of the increase in the level of *cross-linking* and genetic damage to the body's cells which they can bring about.

Cross-linking is an oxidation reaction during which undesirable chemical bonds are formed. It appears to be a major force in body ageing and in the development of a number of degenerative diseases from cancer to arthritis. It's important to know what positive action you can take against environmental threats if you are going to look and feel your very best. Let's look at some of the most important influences and how to counter them.

Life in the Not-So-Great Outdoors

Air pollution, which is widespread in Britain and North America, can be a major obstacle to attaining high-level wellness and to maintaining youthful good looks as the years pass. And, the surprising thing to most people is that the most dangerous airborne pollutants are not contained in the heavy black smoke you see billowing forth from factory chimneys. Like the deadly acid rain, they are virtually invisible to the eye and nose. What's in 'subtly' polluted air? A long list of nasty-sounding substances such as carbon monoxide, benzoprene, tars, ethyl lead and sulphur dioxide which cause nylon hosiery to disintegrate rapidly, deplete your body of important nutrients and even erode the marble and granite of buildings. Modern air pollutants can also cause trouble for skin – or rather *troubles*: dryness, discolourations, and spots, not to mention a lot of more serious conditions from seborrhoea, acne and psoriasis to some elusive forms of contact dermatitis which dermatologists tend to group together under the heading of *dermatitis urbis* – city skin. No matter how fit you are and how well you eat you cannot avoid exposure to toxic metals and other airborne substances which build up in your body and on the surface of your skin to cause trouble. The precise effect of many air pollutants is still unknown. The actions of those which are relatively well understood are enough to make any self-respecting hypochondriac's hair stand on end and to worry even the most conservative 'turn-a-blind-eye' politician. For instance, oxidizing chemicals such as ozone and nitrous oxide in air harm the body in at least two well-proven ways: they cause oxidation reactions in the lungs which can result in lung diseases and reduce your body's ability to get the oxygen it needs from the air, and they destroy vitamin A which is necessary for the health of mucous membrane. Like other gaseous and particulate airborne pollutants they also appear to be major contributors to ageing. The heavy metals are particularly dangerous. Cadmium from cigarette smoke slowly builds up in the system of people exposed to it in offices, restaurants and public places – particularly if you, like many people, are even marginally deficient in one or more of the following nutrients: vitamin B6, zinc, iron, manganese, selenium, calcium, vitamin C or vitamin D. Cadmium levels in tinned food tend to be on the high side, too. When cadmium levels are high enough this can result in adrenal and liver damage and in anaemia.

Other pollutants such as carbon monoxide from car engines, factories and cigarettes replace some of the oxygen in your bloodstream. They can be especially harmful to people with vulnerable lungs or hearts as well as causing headaches and impaired muscle functions even in the most fit and healthy. Environmental lead, which we take in primarily from petrol fumes, can lead to anaemia, kidney, heart and thyroid damage as well as degeneration of the brain. It has even been shown to be responsible for poor learning and behavioural problems in children. And these are only a few of the known environmental threats to health. We are also exposed to insecticides, carcinogenic plastics like PVC, plasticizers such as polychlorinated biphenyls, aluminium from toothpastes, deodorants, antacids and pans we cook in, and a thousand other environmental pollutants. And the United States Surgeon General has stated that the literally hundreds of toxic environmental pollutants to which we are exposed are a major cause of degenerative disease.

Here's the Good News

But there is no reason to brand yourself a victim of your poisonous environment and give up before you start. Nor need you bury your head ostrich-fashion and call it all scare-mongering. There are strong indications that, provided you follow an ultrahealth lifestyle – particularly in its nutritional and fitness aspects – and provided you learn how specific nutrients and other substances can be used to counter the detrimental effects of environmental pollution, you should sail through the turn of the next century laughing. For instance, cadmium toxicity can be prevented by ensuring you get sufficient selenium and zinc in your diet. Experts in trace mineral balance have also shown that cadmium build-up in a body can be removed using iron and vitamin C supplements. There are similar techniques now known for combating the effects of many other major environmental pollutants. Also, a lot of exposure to environmental hazards can be avoided. You can refuse to sit in smoke-filled rooms, you can say no to unnecessary x-rays and you can eliminate carcinogenic plastics from your home and work area. Finally, although governments are notoriously slow even to acknowledge the health dangers implicit in many of the 70,000 to 100,000 chemicals which inhabit our everyday environment, public pressure to improve standards of what constitutes 'pure water', to delineate just what kind and what level of fumes from industry and automobiles we allow to pollute our atmosphere and to stop the dumping of nuclear wastes into our seas which pollute the fish we eat with radioactivity, does eventually get results. A few years ago ministers claimed there were no lead dangers from car exhaust fumes. Now we have unleaded fuel in every petrol station. Pressure from you can help. Political action is an important ingredient in any lifestyle for high-level wellness.

Water Warnings

Natural spring water, laboratory-tested for quality and uncontaminated by chemical additives, is vital for ultrahealth. The water which comes pouring from our taps nowadays is quite different. Far from improving your state of health, it may actually be damaging it. Recent studies show that the water supplies in Europe, North America, Australia, New Zealand and South Africa are freely laced with potentially harmful chemicals. These include pesticides, heavy metals such as cadmium and lead, nitrates, viruses, asbestos, and more than 300 organic chemicals, some of which have already been shown to be cancer-causing. Water in some areas has been linked to a high incidence of death from heart attacks. The presence of high lead levels in water in other areas is now considered responsible for many behavioural problems and cases of low-intelligence ratings in children.

Water has always been something we take for granted. Now such findings are forcing scientists to take a long look at the waters we drink. Few like what they see.

Impossible Task

What is going on? In theory, our governments are obliged to provide pure water. In practice, however, carrying out this obligation is now so costly that no taxpayer would tolerate the burden. As a result of worldwide environmental pollution it would be nearly impossible to implement. Nitrates from our farms, acid rain, weed-killers, fertilizers and pesticides, nuclear wastes and the chemical by-products of runaway industrialization have polluted our rivers, dumps, and land-fill sites. From there they seep back into the water table to show up as far as 100 miles away. Even in the most remote regions of Antarctica man-made chemicals such as the poly-chlorinated biphenyls (PCBs) now pollute fish and wildlife despite their living thousands of miles from the so-called civilized world. Yet the public still remains largely unaware of how bad it has become.

The Clean-Up

The technology we still use for cleaning our water is obsolete. We add chlorine, aluminium and other chemicals as part of the attempt to purify water for drinking. Yet many of the chemicals we still use are themselves pollutants that can make matters worse. Chlorine, which we use to kill bacteria, has been linked to the development of anaemia, high blood pressure, and diabetes. It reacts with industrial effluent polluting our ground water to form cancer-causing compounds. In the United States, where the awareness of these water problems and water treatment itself is believed to be the most advanced in the world, only 50 of the 60,000 public water systems use up-to-date water purification methods. The whole issue of water pollution and the effect it is having on health – yours and mine – is a huge one far beyond the scope of this little book. But what is important is this: if you want a lean, strong, beautiful and healthy body you need to find a source of water that is clean.

This is not an easy task. Most water filters only do part of the job and for any filtering system to work it has to be cleaned and serviced frequently. Boiling your water will kill most bacteria and boil off some of the chlorine but won't move heavy metals and chemical pollutants. Filtering your water through carbon filters will remove pesticides, chlorine and suspended particles, but bacteria from contaminated water poured through them tends to colonize and grow between the carbon particles so they need to be cleaned and changed often. Some manufacturers have added silver to these units to inhibit bacterial growth yet silver itself is a contaminant when taken in quantity. This kind of filter won't touch heavy metals like lead and aluminium which have become *dissolved* in the water.

The effective removal of all impurities from water demands

large, multi-staged and highly complex filter systems operated under carefully controlled conditions. Few home filtering systems (apart from quite costly reverse osmosis units) are capable of removing anywhere near a cross-section of contaminants.

Friends of the Earth will let you have information about how to check out the condition of your own tap water and what your statutory rights are. Put pressure on government and read everything you can on the state of your local and natural water. This is a huge issue for the health of yourself and your family and without massive public pressure unlikely to change. In the meantime take a good look at what inexpensive jug filters are available and start using one – for cooking too. Be sure to change the filter it contains often and regularly. If you can afford it use the best bottled water for drinking.

Drink Your Health

Bottled waters differ tremendously from one to another. Some which come in plastic containers or glass bottles in the supermarket are nothing more than tap water which has been run through conditioning filters to remove the taste while doing nothing to improve the quality. And just because they say 'spring' on the label that doesn't mean a thing. The word may be nothing more than the brand name used to sell the product. Other bottled waters are excellent in taste and quality. Few countries do much to regulate standards for bottled water and what regulation there is is generally even poorer than that applied to tap water. Except in France.

There are some 1,200 springs in France. Several dozen of them supply bottled waters the quality of which has long been monitored and controlled by official government bodies. A few have been granted the title *eau minérale naturelle*. This means that they maintain a constant mineral content. It also means that they have a reputation for specific therapeutic properties. These waters should be safe from bacterial or chemical contamination and you can be sure they have not been mixed with any foreign substance when they are bottled.

Two of the best mineral waters are Volvic, an exceptionally pure still water from the Auvergne mountains in central France, and the sparkling Perrier which arrives in a carbonated form from a spring at Vergèze in Southern France. The Volvic spring is surrounded by seventeen square miles of countryside free from industry, intensive farming and other nearby sources of pollution. Volvic is lightly mineralized with a lot of character and a vibrant quality. The well-known Perrier has long been recommended by French doctors after strenuous exercise. It is a refreshing drink, popular with athletes. I like the taste of it. I also approve of the responsible way in which the Perrier company chose to withdraw hundreds of millions of bottles from the market a few years ago when they discovered that some had been contaminated with benzene from a faulty filter. It showed a sense of responsibility I would like to see copied by other companies. Finally, from the Western region of the Vosges mountains in France comes one of the finest of them all: Vittel Bonne Source. Pure and delicate in flavour, Vittel water wends its way through rock tunnels then pours forth clean and fresh from a source surrounded by 12,000 acres of conservation land in north-eastern France.

Defeat Passive Smoking
Don't let smoke hazards get to you:

- Tell people you live and work with you are bothered by cigarette smoke and ask them please not to smoke.
- Be firm with those that violate no smoking rules on trains and in theatres, etc.
- Sit in non-smoking areas of restaurants, planes and cinemas.
- Make sure any room you're in where people are smoking is well-ventilated.
- Take supplements of the anti-oxidant nutrients such as vitamin C, zinc, betacarotene and the B complex vitamins to protect yourself against smoke hazards.

Cigarettes and Alcohol: Self-Induced Pollution
Almost everybody knows by now that cigarette smoking can cause cancer, heart disease, emphysema, stomach ulcers, and babies of low birth weight born of mothers who smoked during pregnancy. But there are lots of other more subtle ways in which smoking also interferes with high-level wellness. For instance, it suppresses the functions of your immune system because it uses up vitamin C, needed in the body for the leucocytes that act as a mainline defence

against disease. Suppressed immune function makes you highly vulnerable to rapid ageing as well as illness. And just because you yourself don't smoke, don't think you are immune to cigarette-related hazards. Two thirds of the smoke from a cigarette never gets into the lungs of the smoker. Instead it pollutes the environment. You inhale smoke in restaurants, offices and other closed areas. Animal experiments have shown that the noxious substances in this 'secondary' environmental smoke can cause serious illness. It contains many carcinogens such as nitrosamines, nitrogen dioxide, hydrogen cyanide, arsenic and formaldehyde as well as tar and nicotine, carbon dioxide and ammonia. Cigarette smoke is particularly damaging to skin, again because it depletes the system of vitamin C, zinc, and the *bioflavonoids* all of which are needed to make new *collagen* – the structural protein which gives your skin its youthful firmness. If you smoke you should consider taking an extra 10,000 IU a day of betacarotene, a good high-potency B complex vitamin, at least 1,000 mg extra of vitamin C, 100 mg of the bioflavonoids and 12 mg of zinc. If you are really serious about ultrahealth goals, give it up altogether. Bad habits, like unjust rules, are made to be broken. If you are a non-smoker, refuse to let the health-destroying habits of other people impinge on your good looks and vitality by avoiding smoke-filled areas as much as possible.

Get High without Alcohol

Many ultrahealth seekers find that a low-fat diet high in fresh raw fruits and vegetables plus lots of exercise turns even one glass of good wine into a real 'buzz'. Others claim they can get high on mineral water alone. And there are no penalties for drivers caught drinking mineral waters!

The Two Faces of Alcohol

Alcohol is perhaps the strangest of all the pollutants for although it has serious and permanent health-damaging characteristics, in small quantities it may even help protect against heart attacks. A few studies in Europe and America have shown that people who don't take alcohol at all are more likely to suffer a heart attack than those who drink one or more ounces of the stuff a day. Alcohol in small quantities seems to raise the levels of high-density *lipoproteins* in the blood. These blood factors appear to offer some protection against coronary artery disease. A little alcohol – no more than a glass or two of wine a day – also relaxes people and can even improve the digestive system. That is alcohol's smiling, benign face. Its other mask is anything but cheerful.

The Darker Side of Alcohol
Like smoking, alcohol can also cause impaired immunological responses making you more susceptible to infection, early ageing and cancer. More than three drinks a day has been shown to produce liver degeneration, mental disorders and lead to heart disease. Alcohol is also the leading cause of road accidents and fatalities. It's an important cause of birth defects even when a pregnant woman drinks as little as one ounce of it a day. Alcohol is also a common trigger for gout attacks – especially if you consume a lot at one time. It interferes with your sleep by blocking REM dreaming and increasing insomnia. It intensifies depression. Its two-faced nature can be particularly difficult for men in relation to their sexuality. For while consuming alcohol heightens sexual desire because of its stimulating effect on a hormone called LH, it also impairs potency by causing the liver to break down testosterone, the male sex hormone. If you drink long enough and hard enough, the alcohol you consume can chronically lower testosterone levels so that the testicles shrink. Some men in whom this has occurred have even shown signs of female secondary sex characteristics such as breast development.

Drinking alcohol dramatically increases your body's need for many nutrients including the B vitamins such as niacin, thiamine, folic acid and vitamin B6 as well as magnesium, zinc and the essential fatty acids. Because it is a natural diuretic it makes your body lose water from its tissues. Drinking it can deplete your system of many water-soluble minerals, such as potassium, which are important for high-level health. So while the occasional glass of brandy won't hurt you and a glass of wine might even help your digestion, more alcohol than that plays no part in an ultrahealth lifestyle.

Office Pollution is Common
If you find yourself with a headache, chronic tiredness or

mysterious symptoms such as irritated eyes or nose or skin rashes when you are at the office, chances are you are one of a growing number of people suffering from 'indoor climate syndrome' which is a fancy way of saying the effects of office pollution. The symptoms can come from the chemicals and dust of carbonless copy paper and also the radiation from visual display units on word processors or computers and copying machines. Here are some ways of avoiding the problems:

- Don't tear paper or do other things that can create dust in the office and see that it remains as clean as possible.
- Keep copying machines in different rooms from the ones you work in.
- Make sure your office is well ventilated and no hotter than 67 to 68 degrees Fahrenheit.

Radiation, the Silent Menace

Perhaps the most insidious of all the environmental challenges facing high-level wellness is the threat of damage from man-made radiation. It comes in many forms, all of which can be hazardous – from the outpourings of nuclear power plants to simple dental x-rays. What is particularly worrying about radiation is the fact that few people give much thought to how it may be affecting their lives. Marie Curie discovered radium at the beginning of the twentieth century. Years later exposure to it killed her. Radiation is far more dangerous and two-faced than alcohol. We have long known that high levels of radiation can kill. What scientists have discovered more recently is that even very low levels over a long period of time can cause genetic damage to the unborn and produce illness and prematurely age an organism.

What is Radiation?

Radiation is the emission of electromagnetic energy from certain materials into the surrounding medium as they undergo natural changes. Radiation comes in many forms: x-rays, infrared rays, microwaves and others. Some kinds of radiation, such as that caused by atomic fallout, affect the whole body, while the effects of other kinds such as x-rays appear to be confined mostly to specific areas. Intense radiation exposure is a relatively recent but pervasive influence on our environment. It is emitted from our microwave ovens, radios and televisions, power-transmission lines, industrial and military installations, burglar-alarm systems, screening devices at airports and in shops, and medical and dental x-rays – not to mention the kind of nuclear wastes which pollute the fish swimming in our seas, which we eat even if we live far away from nuclear power plants. Scientists measure radiation in rems. Exposure to 100,000 millirems (a millirem is a thousandth of a rem) causes radiation sickness. 500,000 millirems will kill you. But according to a recent report from the National Academy of Sciences Committee on the Biological Effects of Radiation in the United States, genetic damage and cancer occur at far lower levels – levels which had before been considered 'safe'. In fact there appears to be no 'safe' level of radiation. Studies on the effect of simple microwave radiation, such as that generated by a telephone relay system or a television transmitter, show that it can induce changes in the blood-brain barrier and cause central nervous system disorders as well as headaches, fatigue and emotional disturbances. If you live in an urban environment, chances are you are immersed in a complex network of radiation, the damaging effect of which depends mostly on just how well you are able to resist it.

How to Cope with the Radiation Challenge

First, eliminate any unnecessary exposure to radiation in your personal life, and lobby governments to exercise more stringent controls over radiation in your environment. Second, make use of some of the natural protectors against radiation poisoning. Take seaweed, for instance. Studies have shown that the alginate in seaweed or kelp protects an organism from absorbing radioactive Strontium 90, which is in the atmosphere as a result of nuclear fallout and is very dangerous to the body. Among other things, Strontium 90 tends to replace calcium in the bones and to lead to bone disease and cancer. Kelp appears to be helpful in protecting against other kinds of environmental pollutions as well. The fucoidin it contains helps block lead absorption in the body and there is some evidence that, like pectin (a form of dietary fibre which is found in good quantities in apples), it also helps remove much cadmium, aluminium and lead poisoning from the body. Taking kelp tablets daily or eating seaweeds in soups and vegetable dishes or laver bread also helps prevent heavy metal build-up in the first place.

Siegmund Schmidt, the European expert in protecting the body from the hazards of environmental pollution, who is often called on to testify in international court cases in this area, claims that other substances found in foods or taken as nutritional supplements can help enormously too: among them he lists the bioflavonoids, colourants which occur in the whitish flesh of citrus fruits such as oranges, grapefruits and lemons; beetroot and its juice which contain another colourant known to protect against genetic damage in animals; and dry extract of ginseng. Naturally fermented milk products such as yogurt and acidophilus have also been shown to neutralize poisons such as DDT and Strontium 90. So have specially-grown yeast products such as zell-oxygen and Biostrath. Schmidt and others have well documented the protective effects of these factors on animals. They insist that anyone who is concerned with promoting high-level health use them regularly. American expert Dr Carl Pfeiffer adds lecithin to the list of the natural protectors: it neutralizes poisons such as drugs, nitrites, mercury and DDT.

Anti-Pollutant Nutrients

- Vitamin C counters lead build-up in the body and can even gradually eliminate stored lead. It also detoxifies other toxins including cadmium, mercury and many allergens.

- Vitamin A helps protect lung and other tissue from damage caused by oxidizing chemicals in the air.

- Vitamin E acts as an anti-oxidant for the body's lipid-based membranes and increases tissue protection when used with vitamin A. It also protects against carbon monoxide and detoxifies chlorinated pesticides and solvents.

- The alginates – forms of fibre present in seaweeds – help bind heavy metals in the gut (preventing their absorption) and eliminate radiation pollution from the body.

- Selenium has a number of beneficial effects including detoxifying mercury and protecting the body against excess copper and cadmium.

Natural Antidotes to Pollution
Make them an important part of your nutrition lifestyle:

- The bioflavonoids which occur in the white flesh of citrus fruits.

- Naturally fermented milk products such as yogurt and acidophilus cultures.

- Yeast-based products such as zell-oxygen and Biostrath.

- Pectin, a good form of fibre, which occurs in good quantity in apples.

- Lecithin which helps neutralize drugs, nitrites and mercury.

- Beetroot and its juice because of the colourant they contain.

- Kelp and the seaweeds because of the alginate they contain.

Take a Double-Edged Sword to Pollution
So the first hurdle in the ultrahealth game is quite simply life in the twentieth century, with the kind of negative social norms that exert such pressure and all the environmental pollution to which we are exposed. This is compounded by the sedentary lifestyle many people lead (more about that later). The ways of leaping this hurdle, like every hurdle you will come across in playing the ultrahealth game, are twofold:

1. Protect yourself from what hampers your pursuit of personal wellness
and
2. Take an active part in changing the environment in which you and your family live – through increasing your awareness of the extent and effects of environmental hazards – from radiation to agricultural spraying of foods – and then using political pressure to change things for the better. Real health is not a goal that can be pursued in isolation. It demands group effort as well.

PART TWO

BODY POWER

4
Dynamic Fitness Starts Here

THINK OF FITNESS and chances are you think of some 'jock' obsessed with his body – a physical training freak who eats nothing but steak and lettuce leaves and spends hours in front of a mirror admiring his muscles. Not interesting. And *decidedly* not for you. That's how lots of busy people feel about exercise. It is certainly how I used to feel. But dynamic fitness in no way has to include the kind of narcissistic self-watching that a few 'sports nuts' seem to indulge in. Neither will it take away from your aesthetic appreciation of life nor from intellectual pursuits. Most ultrahealth players find it can enhance both, thanks to the biochemical effects that regular vigorous exercise has on the brain. In fact, only when your body is put through its paces and physically challenged can your mind and emotions function at the peaks. For vigorous exercise, like light and air and food, is nothing less than an evolutionary *need* of man. Without constant use your body will not work well, or stay young-looking. Neither are you likely to know just how much creative enjoyment of work and play you are capable of. Exercise – steady rhythmic movement coupled with periods of slow stretching for flexibility – is a major channel to ultrahealth because it is a potent force towards making use of your full potential in every area of your life.

Dynamic Fitness Creates Energy to Spare
Regular vigorous exercise increases rather than depletes your energy. Aerobic activities such as running, brisk walking, steady swimming, dancing, rebounding (on a trampoline) and cycling help your body counter fatigue because they increase your ability to handle a larger workload, both mentally and physically.

Energy for work and for your body's metabolic activities is produced in your muscle cells in little energy factories called *mitochondria*. Here it is stored in the form of adenosine triphosphate (ATP). When your body needs energy to carry out some task like breaking down a protein or producing a hormone or thinking a thought, it calls upon ATP in the mitochondria, rather as you might go to your bank to withdraw cash from an account in order to pay a bill. When you exercise regularly for at least a six-month period important changes take place in your cells. The number of mitochondria in each increases. This creates more sites for the production of the energy-rich ATP so that the total quantity of this compound increases and it is produced much more rapidly than before. This is one of the reasons why people who take up a programme of aerobic exercise report they discover new reserves of vitality. An American professor of physical education, Tom Cureton, surveyed some 2,500 people who took up regular exercise and found that they had significantly more energy and less tension than before, when they led more sedentary lives.

Using Fitness to Alter Paradigms Towards Ultrahealth
Just as we are all strongly influenced by existing social and family 'norms', each of us is governed by personal constructs which consist of ideas we have about reality, notions of how we see ourselves and what we believe to be our strengths and our weaknesses, and how we view the world. Out of such personal constructs we build paradigms about what is possible for us. For most of us these paradigms are narrow. Our view of 'health' is limited to the notion of a state in which we show no overt symptoms of disease. Our vision of ourselves is strongly restricted by whatever limiting ideas we may have such as an unconscious sense that we are basically unworthy. Perhaps you don't strive hard because you believe that you are only capable of achieving so much. Often you don't expect to be really happy, really fulfilled, because you believe (again unconsciously) that, well, that just can't happen to *me*. Or can it?

Contemporary humanistic ideas are founded on the belief that the ultimate mission of human intelligence is the potentiation of self. A broadening of the limits of your paradigms is an important key to this self-fulfilment, and thanks to the intricate relationship between mind and body, one of the most effective ways of enlarging those paradigms – bringing you a sense that many more things are possible than you may before have dreamed of – is regular, vigorous exercise. It is this fact – a discovery made again and again every time a lounge-lizard discovers dynamic fitness – that makes exercise such a central dimension in any ultrahealth lifestyle.

Fitness Brings a New Self-Image

Studies of people who have taken up exercise show that certain very positive psychological changes take place in the way they feel about themselves and their lives and therefore in how effective they are at actualizing their potentials and accomplishing what they set out to do. In part this is to do with biochemical and physiological changes that occur in fitness, in part it is no doubt a simple change in self-image. J. E. Kane, who when he was at London University became well known for his study of the psychological effects of sports, has said: 'The way an individual characteristically perceives his body has long been held as an important factor in forming his image of himself and in his general integration.' This, along with the health-protective benefits of exercise, is why many multi-national corporations have funded programmes of exercise for executives and why so many men and women claim that exercise has helped them to become more effective and to feel more in control of their lives. In an interesting study carried out at Purdue University in the United States, 60 middle-aged people in sedentary jobs participated in a four-month exercise programme which consisted mostly of running. 'Before' and 'after' tests were given to evaluate their personalities. Using the standard Cattel 16 Personality Factor Questionnaire, researchers found these people had become more emotionally stable, self-sufficient, imaginative and confident. Exercisers themselves will tell you that starting on a fitness programme has heightened their mental acuity and improved their concentration, as well as strengthening willpower and increasing their ability to keep going even during extreme fatigue.

Exercise Boggles Your Mind

Dynamic fitness is a total psychosomatic way of being. And exercise as a tool for ultrahealth is not only a matter of achieving a certain level of physical fitness where your heart and lungs work better and you look leaner and firmer. It calls forth or 'turns on' a state of consciousness which is more positive. It dramatically alters your whole outlook on life, bringing you a sense of long-term wellbeing. Depressed people who are put on a programme of regular aerobic exercise a few times a week lose their tendency to become depressed. Such changes make it far easier to follow a lifestyle for ultrahealth. When you feel good and positive about yourself it is easy to forgo foods which are not good for you and you tend to leave behind bad habits. You simply don't want or need them any more.

The biochemical explanation for the kind of positive emotional and mental changes fitness brings currently revolves around messenger chemicals called neurotransmitters which carry powerful implications for mental clarity and moods. Nobel laureate Julius Axelrod, who isolated the neurotransmitter *noradrenaline*, has suggested that a deficiency of this hormone may be the cause of depression. Noradrenaline is known for its ability to lift your mood and to lessen sensations of discomfort and fatigue. (People who are sunny-dispositioned tend to have high levels of noradrenaline in their bloodstream, depressed people have low levels.) Other research has shown that international-class athletes tend to produce high levels of this hormone which appears to help them accomplish supreme feats of endurance. Vigorous exercise enhances the production of noradrenaline. This is probably one of the main reasons why so many emotional disorders, from anxiety to depression, have now been successfully treated with exercise.

Robert Greenwood at the Menninger Foundation has his own idea about why exercise is able so significantly to alter people's moods. Like Kane, he points out that mind distortions are often accompanied by distortions in muscle function. This is one of the reasons mentally-disturbed people often make strange movements with their bodies. He insists that the treatment of emotional and physical disorders must go hand-in-hand and that exercise can play an important part – not only for those severely troubled, but for the average person who is not as positive and not as effective as he or she might be.

Want to Grow Lean?
Then get moving. Animal studies show that sedentary animals eat more than moderately active animals and slowly put on weight. Very

active animals on the other hand consume more food than moderately active ones and still remain lean. The same is true of people. Studies of overweight girls in secondary school show that they actually consume fewer calories than their thin friends. The significant difference is that they are less active physically. Statistics show clearly that a treatment for overweight which relies chiefly on cutting back calories worked in only somewhere between five and twenty per cent of the cases. Add exercise to the regime and effectiveness rapidly and significantly increases. This is not only because physical exertion burns calories (and the calorie-burning factor is *least* important in weight-loss), it is because regular vigorous movement – practised for more than 30 minutes a session, several times a week, increases both metabolic activity and thermogenesis, so that you burn up energy more effectively even when you're resting. This is thanks, at least in part, to increased ATP activity in your cells. For would-be slimmers a religiously-followed exercise programme creates a virtuous circle, reinforcing their commitment to the programme mentally and physically.

Steady vigorous exercise will *not* increase your appetite, as many people believe. It *decreases* it; and its effect on appetite suppression is cumulative so that the longer you continue on your programme the less inclined you will be to overeat. Finally, thanks to its effect on emotions, exercise helps the would-be slimmer improve his or her mental outlook and avoid that 'slump of impossibility' which anyone who has quite a lot of weight to lose knows only too well.

Are You a Fat-Burner?
Short-term exercisers are glucose-burners. They never get their fat supplies to budge. Long-term exercisers – those who spend 45 minutes working out in each session and who work out four to six times a week – burn fat. The enzymes that burn fat are quite different from those that burn glucose. If you are out of shape and fat, your ability to burn fats for energy greatly decreases. The fitter you get, the more fat you will burn. And following the ultrahealth way of eating as well, the thinner you'll become.

Need to Stay Lean?
If you are simply concerned with maintaining the weight you are now you should know that most joggers and runners report they can

eat as much as they like without putting on extra pounds, provided their training is strenuous enough and very regular – several times a week. Running, rebounding, skipping rope, swimming, skiing and rowing are all useful in trimming off weight because they use large muscle groups and because they are both aerobic (they require a steady flow of oxygen) and rhythmical. But to trim pounds off or keep them off if you tend to be a natural weight-gainer, your work-outs need to be *long*. The energy for short periods of high-intensity exercise is derived almost entirely from stored carbohydrates in the muscles and the liver. Only moderately intense activities, such as rebounding or running for *more* than half an hour at a time, will start to burn stored fat. After the first half-hour carbohydrates in the form of *glycogen* in the muscles can contribute no more than half the energy needed to sustain movement so your body is forced to begin releasing its fat stores. To take advantage of this fat-burning ability you need to exercise *at least* three times a week (four or five is much better) for 30 minutes to an hour at a time. Twice-weekly exercise, no matter how intensive or how long, simply doesn't do the trick. Neither will five fifteen-minute sessions.

The Benefits of Regular Workouts

There are now a hundred well-established reasons why exercise is good for you, most of them well documented by research in the expanding field of sports medicine. And most experts agree on these general benefits of regular workouts:

- Increased energy and stamina.

- The replacement of intramuscular fat with lean muscle tissue which produces a more efficient use of calories from the foods you eat. (Most of your calories are burnt off by lean muscle tissue. Nothing is burnt by fat tissue.)

- Improved absorption and improved use of nutrients from the foods you eat.

- Better sleeping habits and more restful sleep.

- Improved self-image, increased good looks and a more positive attitude to life.

- Fewer drugs, and less coffee, tea, and alcohol, refined carbo-hydrates and sugar are consumed by exercisers than by sedentary people.

- Improved emotional state.

- A significant retardation of the ageing process.

- Healthier skin with fewer wrinkles.

Get Moving to Counter Stress
A high level of regular aerobic physical activity burns off a lot of toxic substances taken in from your foods and your environment and eliminates many harmful metabolic wastes which otherwise contribute greatly to a feeling of mental and physical tension and fatigue. It also uses up a number of chemicals produced by your body when it is under stress. So it is one of the very best methods you can find for combating the negative effects of long-term stress, as well as getting rid of that awful pressured feeling which comes when you are worried, overworked or anxious.

When you are under stress, from whatever cause, your body produces a number of chemicals under the direction of the sympathetic branch of your autonomic nervous system. These chemicals are designed to mobilize the body for fight or flight. But, because modern life is so sedentary, most people simply never get a chance to burn them off. For instance, excess adrenaline and its related products tend to get stored in the brain and heart, where they can affect function and alter your responses to things and your moods. Physical activity causes these stored products to be metabolized and clears away the 'adrenaline build-up' which has accumulated from stress. It leaves you feeling relaxed and restores a healthy balance to your autonomic nervous system. It also makes your whole body stronger so that you are more resistant to whatever stressors you happen to come up against. You can then work harder and longer without negative effects.

Exercise Information for 'Disease-Avoiders'
Those are some of the many 'positive reasons' – ultrahealth reasons – why you should make regular exercise a part of your everyday life. There are lots of 'negative' benefits to fitness as well – things which

you protect yourself against if you do. For being inactive is a serious health hazard. It engenders chronic fatigue, high blood pressure, mental inefficiency, premature ageing and stiff or flabby bodies (in some cases both). These conditions in turn are major contributors to injury, tension, overweight, back pain, and heart disease. No matter how well you eat, how much rest you get and how much time you spend looking after yourself, if you don't get enough exercise you cannot be optimally fit or healthy. When it comes to the human body the old adage 'use it or lose it' applies.

Dynamic Fitness Helps Keep You Well

There is a lot of evidence that the effects of regular exercise outweigh even those of a change in diet in the prevention of many diseases, from heart disease to diabetes and even cancer. And this is as true for common acute health problems as it is for serious diseases. Researchers have found that university students who exercise regularly have very few physical complaints while those who don't continue to seek medical help for digestive upsets, fatigue, menstrual problems, backaches, colds and allergies. Both diabetes and hypoglycaemia have been linked to lack of exercise. And exercise can even be instrumental in their cure. One American physician, James Anderson, has shown that diabetics with blood sugar counts as high as 350 (just below 100 is normal) can often be freed from dependence on drugs by taking regular exercise. And of course the protection which being active offers against heart disease (regardless of what other 'risk factors' – such as cigarette smoking, high blood pressure, and parental heart attacks – may be present) has been well established.

Nutritional Supplements and Athletics

- 84 per cent of Olympic athletes rely on nutritional supplements to strengthen their performance. The requirements for some vitamins and minerals increase when you exercise a lot.

- Winning athletes have higher vitamin B1 intakes than losing ones, and some athletes claim extra B1 helps fight fatigue in marathons.

- Vitamin B3 and vitamin B12 work in synergy with B1.

- Vitamin C helps the body burn its free fats as energy, benefits oxygen metabolism and may also increase adrenaline production during exercise.

Any supplements you take to improve athletic performance need to be supported by the full range of nutrients including vitamins A, E, D and the rest of the B group to be effective. They all work together.

How Exercise Looks After Your Heart

Any kind of aerobic activity which you practise daily or at least several times a week makes your heart work more efficiently. Your heart gradually gets stronger so that it can pump more blood with less effort. And, just as with practice you can exercise for longer periods because your heart is more resilient, so too can you respond better to day-to-day emotional or mental crises without making your heart pound or raising your blood pressure. Vigorous exercise also helps prevent heart disease by developing collateral circulation – new blood vessels which take the burden off long-standing circulation pathways, many of which may have become plaque-choked. This is one reason why patients who, after a heart attack, enter a graded exercise programme have a much better survival rate. Exercise also lowers blood pressure by inducing vasodilatation of muscle arteries and increases the ability of your body to dissolve any clots which may form, thanks to its positive influence on the concentration of lipids in the blood. Recent medical theories indicate that there is an inverse relationship between *high-density lipoproteins* (HDL) and heart disease. People who exercise regularly have significantly higher levels of HDL, which appears to help protect them from heart disease and lower levels of *low-density lipoproteins* (LDL), which are associated with greater risk. And, although as yet there is no absolute proof, many scientists believe that regular exercise may even promote the regression of the *atheromatous process* whereby the arteries become coated with plaque and harden – one of the prime causes of death among western races.

Will Exercise Rejuvenate You?

There is a lot of evidence that it will, quite apart from the fact that it will make you look better and feel firmer. Old people put on a seven-week exercise programme are able to gain a level of fitness comparable to those twenty or twenty-five years younger, regardless of what their health is like at the start of the programme. They lose body fat and gain muscle, their blood pressure is lowered and they have increased oxygen consumption. (A decrease in oxygen consumption and in your body's ability to deliver sufficient blood and oxygen to muscles and tissues to keep skin glowing, eyes bright and all the body's cells functioning well, is just one of the many age-related factors which exercise can reverse.) Exercise also prevents the demineralization of bones known as osteoporosis, which used to be considered an inevitable consequence of getting older. Now we know that it is inactivity rather than age which brings it about. Like many of the so-called characteristics of ageing, it is anything but inevitable and can be prevented – if only you use your body enough.

In fact, disuse – the sedentary life – is responsible for many age-associated changes which exercise can prevent or ameliorate, from varicose veins to chronic digestive disorders. Regular exercise does wonderful things for your skin – athletes have skin significantly younger than non-athletes their age – and for your sex life. It also improves sleep. And there are a number of studies which now show that regular exercise (provided it is *moderate*) makes you live longer. And because of the way in which regular exercise maintains peripheral circulation and optimum oxygenation of the tissues, it combats the development of many circulatory problems characteristic of ageing.

Use It or Lose It
After 24 hours of inactivity your muscle tissue begins to deteriorate. Only regular exercise – both aerobic and weight-bearing exercise such as working out with dumb bells and bar bells – can prevent this. It makes your body change slowly and prevents muscle shrinkage which in turn keeps levels of hormones high – important for youthful skin and healthy sexuality.

Being Fit is Fun
But you want to know the best reason of all to get out and get moving? It's that being fit can be a real joy. Exercise is a lot more than just something you do to stem a spreading waistline. Once you

get used to a regular aerobic routine, the impetus to continue comes from *within,* not from some kind of self-righteous feeling that you *should.* Over a period of several months this kind of exercise opens up a new sense of fun and pleasure about living which makes a lot of things that seemed impossible before possible now. That's the main reason fitness is so important for ultrahealth – it's a key to the unfolding of your potential in all areas of your life. You rediscover how to play – something most of us have forgotten by the age of 10. This play approach to exercise is important to overall wellness in other ways. Two studies in England and Ireland have shown that where hard labour did not alter coronary risk factors in more than 30,000 men, hard physical activity taken for pleasure by the same men in their leisure hours significantly reduced the risks and the number of heart attacks they suffered. The difference was not in the greater physical effort made. The physical effort was the same. It lay in the fact that one activity was *work* – imposed from the outside on the men – and the other *play* – something they took up themselves for their pleasure and benefit.

5
Get Ready

What is Fitness Like?

WHEN YOU ARE really fit you will be strong, supple and have stamina. Strength is muscle power – the extra push that makes you able to deal with unexpected heavy tasks like pushing a car or lifting a heavy load. Suppleness is flexibility, the ability to bend and stretch freely without pain and to twist and turn as you wish. Being supple is being mobile, so you can reach up high for things on a shelf, squat down easily, or sit comfortably in a chair or on the floor for long periods. Your body will stay supple if you use all of its muscles and joints regularly. If you don't you will get stiff and feel old. The notion that because you may be approaching forty or fifty or sixty you can *expect* to get stiff is nonsense. Stiffness at any age can be prevented through a diet low in fat and moderate in protein and high in fresh raw foods, combined with proper exercise. And what is stamina? It's endurance, staying power, the ability to work hard and long without fatigue – not only physical stamina, but mental and emotional stamina too. In order to build both strength and stamina you need to put your body's large groups of muscles – those muscles in your legs and arms for instance – through their paces and to challenge your heart and lungs.

What Kind of Exercise is Best?

There are two basic kinds of exercise: *isometric* and *isotonic*. Isotonic – often called aerobic – exercise is the foundation of dynamic fitness. It involves rhythmic movements of your arms and legs and a shortening and lengthening of these large muscle groups. It also puts your body under measured steady stress which builds its strength, stamina and endurance. Rebounding, running, jogging and aerobic calisthenics or dance are examples of such exercise. So are swimming, cycling and rowing – all of which are known as aerobic activities since they require large amounts of oxygen and because they make your heart work hard to pump a great deal of blood. Their main object is to increase the maximum amount of oxygen your body can process in a given time. This measurement is technically known as your aerobic capacity. It depends on how well your body can take in volumes of air and deliver blood and oxygen to all its parts. Since your aerobic capacity reflects the conditions of your heart and lungs, experts agree that it is the best indicator of overall fitness.

The other main type of exercise is isometric. It is the kind of exercise done without causing much actual movement to take place. Muscle tension exercises done against a wall or desk and some kinds of weight-lifting are examples of this kind of exercise. Tensing muscles as you do in these activities causes them to increase in size and density, since whenever any muscle is placed repeatedly under tension it gradually gets bigger. This is why body builders rely so much on isometrics. But contracting muscles in this way tends to cause blood pressure to rise in some people. Isometrics can help build dynamic fitness. But most importantly, you must go aerobic.

Get into Stretching Too

An aerobic activity is not enough on its own (unless you choose swimming, which is remarkable in that it stretches muscles all over as well as strengthening them). You will need to do a few slow stretching exercises for increasing the flexibility of your joints and balancing the muscle work you are doing. Then you will have an unbeatable combination for long-term good looks, health and vitality. The whole lot should take you 30 to 50 minutes three to six times a week. And just in case you don't think you can find time for exercise – you don't *find* time, you *make* it. But the time you make is never wasted, for it will bring you such rewards in increased energy, mental clarity and fitness that you will more than make up for it in what you accomplish during the rest of your day.

Check on Fitness
To help determine just how fit you are at the present moment here is a little check list. See to how many of the questions below you can answer yes and to how many no.

- Do you tire after carrying a couple of bags of shopping for fifteen minutes?
- Does your heart thump when you climb a flight of stairs?
- Do you suffer aches and pains all round when you dig in the garden?
- Are you tired after eight hours of mental work?
- Are you very tired after two hours of housework or gardening?
- Do you tend to avoid physical effort if you can?
- Are you left gasping for breath if you run a short distance?
- Is it difficult to stretch up to reach for something on a high shelf or to bend over to tie a shoe?
- Do you frequently suffer back pain?

If your answer is yes to any of these questions, more exercise will positively benefit you. If you answered no to all of them then you are probably already fairly fit and can try the more advanced fitness test (see page 59).

Forget the Jock Image
You certainly don't have to be an athlete to achieve a high level of fitness and health. In fact, studies show that the excessive training and stress to which the athlete subjects his body can be counter-productive. 'As far as health is concerned', says Scandinavian expert Per-Olaf Astrand, 'it is not the absolute amount and volume of training that is important but the work in relation to the individual's capacity. The severe, prolonged training of the top athlete adds no health benefits to those of a submaximal training programme twice a week.' Indeed, excessive exercise can under-mine immunity, cause loss of muscle from bones and make you age rapidly. When it comes to using exercise to promote ultrahealth, the goal is not to become a 'sports nut' but just to create an active lifestyle for yourself and then to stick to it. Neither do you need a lot of special equipment. Exercise has become the latest and greatest commodity in our consumer-fixated culture and the exercise

industry (which is one of the fastest growing) is becoming highly sophisticated, selling exorbitantly expensive paraphernalia from computerized bicycles to automatic treadmills and trendy gear to make you *look* athletic. You require none of them to get the benefits of fitness. All that is really needed is motivation, some active involvement and a determination to rearrange your lifestyle so you can fit it all in.

How Fit Are You?

It is important to determine your general level of fitness before you begin any exercise programme, not only to ensure that it is safe for you to take up, but also because the programme you choose will depend on how much fitness is already there.

Try walking up and down a flight of 15 steps quickly three times. If you are reasonably fit you should be able to do this without becoming breathless. If you do become breathless after only one, don't continue – you must be *very* careful to start any new programme for exercise at a basic level and go slowly.

The Principle of Overload

The benefits of exercising come as a result of developing strength by progressively *overloading* your body's muscles (overloading in this context means pushing them beyond the normal work they do). Fitness tests are only useful as a rough gauge to determine your present aerobic capacity and therefore just how much *effort* you will need to make to continue to increase your fitness. It is important to grasp the difference between *work* and *effort*. Two people may run a mile in, say, ten minutes and do equal work. But if one raises his heart-rate by 60 per cent above what it was in a resting state and the other only by 30 per cent then their effort has been different. The heart has had to make a smaller proportional response to the load of exercise because of its efficiency. Effort in this sense means the *effort* your heart is making in response to the *work* your body is doing. In order to build dynamic fitness you have to keep up a certain level of effort for a certain length of time. The amount of work you will have to do to achieve this – the distance you will have to cover and the speed at which you will have to run (or swim or cycle or row) will constantly alter as you get fitter.

Do You Need an ECG Test?

The Royal College of Physicians and the British Cardiac Society state that 'most people don't need a medical examination before starting an exercise programme. There are no risks in regular rhythmic exercise as long as the programme begins gently and only gradually increases in vigour.' But before embarking on any vigorous exercise programme you should consult your doctor (they advise) if:

- You suffer from bronchitis, asthma or other chest troubles or chest pain.
- You have ever had heart disease or high blood pressure.
- You are still recuperating from a recent illness.
- You have dizzy spells or often feel faint.
- You have joint problems such as arthritis.
- You have frequent oedema (water retention) at ankles and/or wrists.
- You are concerned that exercise might affect your wellbeing in any other way.

What to Expect if You Do Have a Medical

There are specific tests which attempt to determine your suitability for an exercise programme. They are usually available in sports medicine clinics and include an examination of your cardiovascular system, muscles and joints. Your blood is analysed for *cholesterol* and *triglycerides* and your blood pressure is taken. A resting ECG is usually given and sometimes the ECG stress test where you pedal a stationary bicycle (a bicycle ergometer) or walk or run on a treadmill in the laboratory or where you climb up and down on a bench while ECG equipment monitors your heart. You may also be asked to breathe into a one-way valve which tells the doctor or physiologist how much oxygen is used during the activity you are performing. This oxygen is measured in litres per minute and then expressed as millilitres of oxygen per kilo of total body weight. The oxygen-count gives the tester a fairly accurate measurement of your aerobic capacity – the rate at which you use oxygen. This kind of testing is particularly useful if you are recovering from a heart attack or you are very unfit to begin with.

But quite apart from their expense and the fact that they are not widely available on the National Health, some studies show also that under the stressful conditions of laboratory testing even healthy people who are quite fit can show up so-called abnormal results.

Alternative Ways of Determining Fitness

A number of researchers have worked to discover simpler ways to test cardio-respiratory endurance and to measure fitness levels based on how quickly your heart recovers after exercise. Some physiology laboratories measure the heart-rate twice – immediately on stopping and then again two or three minutes later. Such a measurement doesn't tell you much, however, because the critical period of recovery is actually in the first minute after the end of exercise. Measuring your heart recovery rate immediately on stopping your activity and then exactly one minute afterwards will give you a far better indication of your fitness level. Your recovery rate is pretty easy to measure for yourself once you get the hang of it.

Here's How: After exercising for five or ten minutes take your pulse immediately by placing three fingers of one hand on the underside of the opposite wrist until you feel a throb. (It can take a bit of practice, but it is very easy to locate the artery with a couple of tries.) Count your pulse for 15 seconds and multiply by 4 to give you your minute pulse-rate. Take your pulse again *exactly* one minute later and again record your minute pulse-rate. Now subtract the second number from the first to get your recovery rate and indicate your level of fitness.

Recovery Rate Formula: Immediate Pulse – 1 Minute Pulse =
Recovery Rate ÷ 10 = Level of Fitness

If the number you get is high then your heart is recovering well and is strong. For instance, if your immediate pulse was 140 beats per minute and 1 minute later it was 100 then $140 - 100 = 40$. $40 ÷ 10 = 4$. This is an indication of a good level of fitness.

Here is a little table to help you measure your fitness.

Less than 2	Poor
2–3	Fair
3–4	Good
4–6	Excellent
More than 6	Superb!

6
Go For It

UNTIL QUITE RECENTLY in human history you simply *had* to be fit or you would not have survived. The life led demanded physical work, movement and activity. The idea of going out for a run or skipping rope would have seemed absurd to someone who spent 14 hours a day in hard labour tilling a field or hunting or protecting his property from possible threats. Now however, immersed in our world of cars and automation, most of us have to make a conscious effort to use our bodies vigorously. We also have to decide, given the kind of life we lead, our preferences and our purse, what kind of aerobic activity is best to pursue.

Which Exercise Is For You?
Most experts agree that, overall, swimming is best, since it is the only form of exercise which develops stamina, strength and suppleness equally well. It is also ideal for anyone overweight or very unfit to begin with, since your body weight is supported by water so there is no extra strain. When it comes to building firm limbs and a strong heart there is nothing like slow steady aerobic swimming for 30 to 40 minutes three or more times a week. But not everybody has easy access to a pool. Also, one of the disadvantages of swimming, especially for women, is the way it can leave your hair in a mess afterwards. Rowing, cycling, jogging, running, aerobic dance and calisthenics or even brisk walking are also good for strength and stamina, but if you choose one of them you will need to do a few slow stretching exercises to help with suppleness. Cycling does not make the demands on the body that running or rowing do, so it can be very good for real beginners too. If you choose it you will

have to cycle for half as much time again as you would run or row or swim in order to get the same workout. In many ways running or jogging (the second is simply a slightly slower version of the first) are the easiest of all the aerobics. You can do them anywhere and anytime with no special equipment but a pair of good running shoes. Also, with running, as your state of fitness increases you can easily increase your speed and/or the length of your runs to keep up with your new stronger, fitter body. My favourite of all forms of aerobic exercise, especially for beginners or people who are overweight, is rebounding – using a mini-trampoline. Still little known, it is a wonderful way of toning up your whole body. It greatly improves lymphatic drainage, eliminates wastes from your system efficiently and leaves you feeling great.

Work Out Regularly

If you can't exercise regularly, you're better off not exercising at all. Working out at weekends or whenever you feel the urge is potentially dangerous, especially if you are over forty, for your head may not be strong enough to withstand erratic strenuous workouts. If you are ill or extremely fatigued it is all right to suspend your exercising temporarily, but regularity (at least two, preferably four or five times a week) is essential for you to hold on to the benefits exercise will bring you. If you don't continue working out this frequently, you will lose what you have gained in terms of dynamic fitness.

Discover the Fun of Rebounding

This consists of movements such as skipping, jumping, running on the spot or arm flinging on a firm mini-trampoline called a 'rebound exercise unit'. Rebounding will do all that other forms of aerobic exercise can – strengthening your heart and lungs and firming your muscles – and more, because of the unique way in which your body is subjected to the changing force of gravity when it bounces up and down. Rebounding crosses the generation gap too. It can be done as easily and as effectively by the sixteen-year-old as it can by an ailing sixty-year-old whose muscles and joints have long ago lost their capacity for smooth movement. Some top athletes use rebounders as part of their training programme, while the old or infirm are given rehabilitation on the same kind of bouncing devices. It all depends on how you use the equipment.

The units, which look rather like low coffee-tables, consist of a steel or aluminium frame on six or eight legs over which is sprung a drum of firm but elastic material on which you bounce. They sit somewhere between six and ten inches off the floor and come in many different sizes and shapes – oval, round, polygonal, square. They don't really seem out of place in the corner of a kitchen or tucked away in the bedroom. In fact, you can use a bouncer anywhere. And people who dislike the rigmarole of changing, running and showering, or who find exercise 'too boring for words' can do their bouncing at home (even with small children running around). With rebounding you can dress in any way you like, watch television, listen to music or carry on a conversation while you are exercising.

Manipulating the Force of Gravity

From a physiological point of view, what gives rebounding its potency for building fitness, improving health and retarding ageing is the way it makes use of the force of gravity. It is the only form of overall vertical, rather than horizontal, exercise anywhere. The upward and downward movement on a bouncer, coupled with acceleration-deceleration, brings about continual changes in the force of gravity exerted on your body. All its organs, the circulatory and lymphatic systems, and even individual cells are affected, in a way that no other form of exercise can accomplish. When running or skipping on a unit, the G-force at the top of the bounce is non-existent, as, for a moment, your body takes on the total weightlessness of an astronaut in space. Then when you come down again onto the elastic mat the pull of gravity is suddenly increased to two or even three times the usual G-force on earth. This puts all parts of your body, from the tiniest cell to the longest bone, under rhythmic pressure.

The kind of cellular stimulation the body receives from this continual gravity/non-gravity exposure appears to have remarkable and unique benefits. Waste materials in cells are gently eased out into the interstitial fluid to be carried through the lymph system and eliminated from the body. Increased oxygen is brought to the cells to stimulate cell metabolism. Cell walls appear to grow stronger and cells to function more efficiently with repeated use of a rebounder. This leads to a gradual detoxification of your whole system, much like that which comes through controlled fasting. The texture of your skin improves, your energy levels rise and sometimes even within only a few days your body begins to look younger and to feel far better. And because rebounding is amusing, it is a form of exercise which even lounge-lizards usually like. Taking it up one week doesn't usually mean giving it up the next. This fun aspect of rebounding can have important implications for anyone wanting to use aerobic exercise to lose excess pounds or look and feel better rapidly with the minimum of effort, as some interesting studies in the United States showed.

Bounce Your Way to a Lean Body

James R. White, a researcher in rehabilitation at the University of California at San Diego, designed an interesting study in the long-term effectiveness of weight-loss programmes using exercise. He put some people on rebounders. Others rode bicycles: some ran on a treadmill. The control group did nothing except diet. All who exercised aerobically lost a significant amount of weight and showed a definite increase in the level of their fitness. But in the follow-up study designed to test long-term effectiveness, only 5 per cent of the cyclists and 31 per cent of the runners were still exercising, while a sound 58 per cent of the bouncers were still bouncing. It helped them remove and keep off the excess pounds. The explanation bouncers gave for continuing to exercise was simple. First, it was easy. Second, it was fun.

Rebounding for Rehabilitation

A number of researchers have shown that using a bouncer regularly can be an excellent way of exercising if your body has sustained some kind of injury, such as a twisted knee or *achilles tendonitis*, while running or doing some other form of exercise. It gives the exercise enthusiast a chance to maintain fitness and still let the injury heal, and helps to avoid the familiar depression that sets in when you cannot exercise. Indeed many exercise physiologists insist that, because of the way in which rebounding affects the body at a cellular level, it can be a significant positive force in encouraging healing, both of minor injuries and of degenerative conditions such as arthritis. At Elks Hospital, Idaho, Dr. Kenneth Smith, Head of the Department of Rehabilitation, reports success in using rebounders when rehabilitating patients with orthopaedic or neurocircular conditions. In a large study involving 2,300 patients in California, in which rebounding was used as the major form of physiotherapy, researchers reported excellent results. Bouncing strengthened muscles, eliminated and prevented pain in the lower back and elsewhere was helpful in treating both osteo- and rheumatoid arthritis.

Getting Started

Whatever aerobic activity you choose – swimming, rowing, cycling, dancing, running, rebounding or any of the others – the important thing is to find the way of fitting it into your life and get busy doing it. (See Chapter 23 for help with that.) Once you have got your routine worked out it is relatively easy to monitor your progress and know when you have to increase your effort to get the workout you need to reach a higher level of physical fitness. You'll be surprised how quickly this happens. Regardless of the kind of aerobics you are doing, the principles are the same. You need to exercise *at least* three times a week for *at least* half an hour at a time and if possible five or six times a week.

Go Easy

If you find that you rated poor on the endurance test (page 57), then you will need to start very slowly. Swimming perhaps, or walking, or gentle rebounding. Then you can gradually increase the intensity of your activity to keep your heart-rate at the level which is optimal for you.

Training Heart-Rate is the Key

Whatever form of aerobic activity you choose it should raise your heart-rate to 60–75 per cent of maximum. This figure, your 'training heart-rate', is easy to determine. In his excellent book on exercise, *Fit or Fat*, the exercise specialist Covert Bailey describes the way to go about it:

• Find your Resting Heart-Rate
Three or four times a day, while you are sitting quietly, take your

pulse-rate on the artery near the base of your thumb at your wrist for 15 seconds. Multiply this figure by 4 to get your resting pulse-rate. Add up the figures for several readings collected during the day and divide by the number of readings you have made to get your average resting heart-rate. Then write it here:

• Calculate your Maximum Heart-rate
To do this simply subtract your age from 220. This figure will give you an indication of the fastest your heart can safely beat at your age. (You must *never* exercise at this level!) Write it here:

• Your Training Level
Now you can calculate your training heart-rate – the ideal level at which your heart should beat while you are carrying out your biogenic exercise activity. You *could* simply work out 75 per cent of your maximum heart-rate, but because you are an individual with individual needs you should calculate a more accurate training heart-rate by subtracting your resting heart-rate from your maximum heart-rate, multiplying by 0.65 (i.e., taking 65 per cent of it) and then adding the result back onto your resting heart-rate again. This will give you your training level – the figure you need to remember and to which you must work. Write it here:

• Example
If you are 45 years old and have a resting heart-rate of 70, then the calculations for your training level would go like this:

$$220 - 45 = 175 \ (175 - 70) \times 0.65 = 68.25$$
$$68.25 + 70 = 138.25$$

In this case your training level should be below 138 (say 140 for convenience) beats a minute for you to get maximum benefits from your exercise. So when you actually are doing your exercise – walking or rebounding or steady swimming or whatever – stop and check your pulse for 15 seconds and multiply by 4 to see that it is at this level. If it is 10 beats per minute (bpm) slower, then you need to make more effort. If it is 10 bpm faster, slow down – you are working too hard and not getting your full fat-burning benefits from the activity.

What to Expect

Once you start any aerobic exercise programme some interesting changes take place. For instance, some people feel fatigued both mentally and physically for a few days. This is because the 'power curve' of muscular strength doesn't rise in a linear way on starting a programme of vigorous exercise. It takes time for your body to adjust to the unaccustomed workload – usually about a week – so that you are in a 'get worse before you get better' situation. It is good to keep this in mind, since knowing it may happen will help keep you from becoming discouraged if it does, and prevent you from leaving off your programme before it begins to show benefits.

The more you exercise, the better your condition will become and the greater will be the rewards. From the first session you will experience a feeling of satisfaction plus a few aches and pains here and there. Very soon, however, you will get into the flow of things and by the end of your first 10 days or two weeks you'll find your energy levels steadily rising and your body feeling great. After three months on your new programme you will probably find you don't want to miss a session because you just won't feel the same if you do. As one physician who uses jogging to treat his patients says, it becomes a 'positive addiction'. Some people even claim to experience a 'high' after completing their usual jog.

The Warm-Up

It is important to begin any aerobic exercise (except swimming) with a 5 to 10 minute period of slow, rhythmic stretching exercises. There is less chance of injuring a muscle if it is thoroughly warmed – indeed, no dancer would go on stage without a thorough warm-up. Doing some warm-up stretching before setting out is particularly important as you get older. Then, not only do one's muscles tend to be stiffer and joints creakier, but studies show that in some people a condition where not enough blood gets to the heart can occur if they launch into vigorous exercise without going through a preliminary warm-up first. Stretching exercises not only have a prophylactic effect on your heart, they also increase your flexibility and help strengthen muscles which you are not using in your aerobic activity. And a good warm-up invigorates your body and gets you into the right frame of mind for your exercise. Do your warm-up in your exercise gear. The stretches should be done gently and slowly so your body gradually becomes warm, yet you are not exhausted at the end of them. Here's how:

The Limbering
Part of the warm-up is directed at stretching the muscles at the back of your legs, and strengthening those in your abdomen and calves. These are particularly important for joggers and cyclists. So the exercises fulfil a double purpose by getting you warm and relaxed while stimulating the heart and lungs and filling in any 'muscle-toning gaps' your aerobic activity creates. Do them *slowly* to prevent opposing muscles contracting too much, and do them *gently* so you never damage tendons.

Back Leg Stretchers
Sit on the floor with your legs slightly bent and lean forward to grasp both ankles. (See that your ankles remain flexed so that your toes are pulled up towards your torso.) Now gently push your ankles with your hands, bending at the hips and bringing your torso and head forward so you straighten your legs as much as possible by sliding your feet along the floor. Don't strain. You can aim to touch your knees with your forehead but it doesn't matter much if you never make it. It is the slow gentle stretch that counts. Now, pulling on your ankles, slowly return to starting position. Repeat 10–30 times, increasing the number as you get fitter. You'll notice your thighs becoming firmer.

Special Sit-Ups
Lie on your back, knees bent and feet flat on the floor. Now with your hands clasped behind your head raise your torso 6–8 inches off the floor (no more) slowly and smoothly. Then slowly and smoothly return to your starting position. These sit-ups are specially designed to bring into play your abdominal muscles which don't get a full workout in the conventional sit-ups where you are lying with legs stretched out which tends to put too much strain on the back. Repeat 15 times and work up gradually to about 50 times.

Foot Twists
Sit in a chair and cross your legs so one leg hangs free. Twist the foot at the ankle round slowly in a clockwise direction, pulling hard

so that the ankle is flexed at the top of the circle and the toes are pulled up hard. If you do it correctly it is quite a difficult exercise. Now reverse the movement and do it counter-clockwise. Then change legs and repeat. This exercise strengthens the front of the legs and the ankles. Do 5–8 circles in each direction for each foot.

Cooling Off

Just as you need to warm up before exercising aerobically, you need to cool your muscles off gradually too. While you are exercising much of your body's blood rushes into the area of muscle you are using. With each movement the contractions in these muscles send the blood rushing back to the heart and the rest of the body. But if you suddenly stop moving, much of the blood can 'pool' in one part instead of being sent back to the brain and the heart. This can result in dizziness, nausea and even more serious problems. You need to take five minutes at the end of your run during which you slow down to a walk but keep moving in order to help eliminate the waste products of exercise quickly and lessen or prevent the heavy, slightly sore, feeling that can follow it. Especially at the beginning – before you are really fit.

In addition to this slow-down period of walking at the end of a run there are some other excellent stretching exercises which are particularly good for hips and legs and will help you develop more flexibility of movement all round:

Side Lunges

Standing with your feet wide apart, hands on hips, bend your left knee, and keeping your right leg straight, press the inside of the right leg towards the ground. Return to starting position. Repeat ten times then change sides.

Forward Lunges

Hands on hips, feet slightly apart, one in front of the other, stretch as far as you can, pressing your bottom forward towards the ground and bending the knee in front of you as you lunge forward. Repeat ten times returning to the starting position each time. Change legs and repeat.

Thinking Positively

Nothing can ruin an exercise programme faster than old-fashioned negative attitudes. Yet many of us are stuck with them because we have grown up to consider exercise something you only do under duress in school or because we believe that exercise is something for fitness freaks or horses – not for us. Although most people have been conditioned like this, anyone who has tried rebounding, or running, or aerobic dance, or swimming, or cycling, or rowing, and come to love it, will tell you that not one of these common notions is true. Exercise is fun. Not at first maybe, for it can be hard work when your muscles are soft, your joints stiff and your heart and lungs not used to so much exertion. At first it is natural to feel a little awkward and heavy, and to wonder how anybody could consider something which takes so much effort a pleasure. But each time you start to work out, instead of harping on the effort involved to get creaky joints moving, let your mind play over all the benefits which it will bring you. You'll find that any original discomfort passes quickly if you just persevere. Remember that many other 'doubters' have already discovered a new, healthier and more exciting way of living through dynamic fitness. Expect this for yourself and you won't be disappointed.

Freshening Up

Once you have cooled off a bit and stopped sweating you will probably want a shower – more invigorating than a bath – but don't make it too hot and try to finish off with a 30-second cold shower.

If you choose to have a bath, be sure the water is warm, not hot. Never soak in really hot water, otherwise you may start sweating again and will feel lifeless and dried up when you get out. When you have washed, try emptying your bath and then refilling it to about eight inches with cold water. Stand in it and sponge yourself down starting with your lower legs and working up to the waist. Then sit down and splash thoroughly your torso and finally your shoulders, neck and head. Finish off with a Turkish towel rubdown and dress warmly afterwards. Cold water used in this way has an exciting effect on the body. It benefits both blood and circulation, and it tones and promotes the repair of muscles. It also makes you feel really good.

PART THREE

HIGH-ENERGY NUTRITION

7
Eating for Vitality

TAKE A LOOK at *why* you eat. Are you one of a small minority of people who eat just to stay alive but have no real interest either in the taste or the health effects of foods? Is your prime interest in diet from an eating-to-stay-thin point of view? Or do you find yourself worrying most of the time about what and how much you eat so you don't get fat? Another motivation when it comes to food is the Dionysian one – choosing foods entirely because they titillate your palate. This is perhaps the most common of all reasons for making dietary choices. Are you a Dionysian eater? Or perhaps, more concerned about health, you are one of a growing number of people who eat to avoid disease? They worry about eating eggs or butter because of the cholesterol these foods contain. These people continually readjust their eating habits to fall in line with the latest medical report on heart disease or cancer. Are you a 'disease-avoider'?

Of course all of us are to some extent influenced by most of those food-motivations at one time or another. But to play the ultrahealth game well, all of the above reasons for choosing foods (including those of the disease-avoiders) need to become subservient to one simple goal: eating for performance and energy. The ultrahealth eater chooses foods both because they look and taste delightful and because they are part of a whole life-enhancing, energy-creating experience. In short, you eat because it makes you feel – and, as a corollary, look – great.

For most people this means making a few changes. And changing your eating habits is almost always a slow process, one in which you take three steps forwards only to follow them with two more backwards. But this kind of slow change tends to be far more permanent than throwing over everything you are used to in favour of whole new habits just like that. The eating goal for ultrahealth is *eventually* to come to like, want and delight in the foods which will do you the most good anyway – not because medical research shows that rats living on them stay healthier. You come to prefer them because they work best for your body and mind and because, instead of robbing your body of vitality as many foods can, they energize you, help to keep you calm in the face of stress, and encourage your body to function in optimal ways, all at the same time. Such is the power of the ultrahealth way of eating. It is a nutritional lifestyle which focuses on the peaks and chooses your eating habits from there. And it demands two things: first, an examination of your own nutritional ways of living now, and secondly, the gradual development of a new nutritional lifestyle which works specifically for you. After a while this new lifestyle becomes second nature. Then you can forget the notions of how much heart disease will be caused in ten years if you do or do not eat that extra egg. Eat so you can bring about optimal energy and functioning in your body and clarity in your mind, and disease-prevention will take care of itself. Look for positive returns from your diet now and you won't have to worry about the future.

Basically you need three diet skills in the ultrahealth game:

- A real desire to kick the junk-food habit.

- A fundamental knowledge of nutrition to the degree that you know what kind of foods are health-enhancing and what kind tend to be health-deteriorating.

- A desire to refocus your food preferences in favour of the former. Making ultrahealth changes in diet are simply not that difficult provided you act on what you learn. Knowledge without action will get you nowhere.

Why is it So Hard to Change Your Way of Eating?
Because the way you eat is the way you have been brought up to eat. It's the way your parents eat, or the way people around you eat. As such it carries with it a whole ethos of belonging, of social patterning and social norms which have a strong hold on most of us. 'Food',

like 'Mother' and 'God', are concepts we all tend to defend irrationally, believing somehow that to change our dietary habits would be to lose a sense of who we are. This is generally more true of men than women. Men I have known have sometimes actually felt unloved if their wives did not provide them with the gravy-laden roast beef and mashed potatoes their mothers used to serve.

Then too, there is the powerful lobbying of our high-technology food industry and the effects of advertising on us. Most people for instance believe that milk is a health-giving, almost *virtuous* drink, for it has been toted to us in that image for the past fifty years. Yet milk has many negative qualities that are usually overlooked. It tends to be mucous-forming, is very high in fat and can be very difficult to digest. Also, many people, whether they know it or not, have lactose-intolerance – an inability to break down the milk sugar in pasteurized milk. When they drink milk their abdomen can become bloated and often very painful or they can be plagued by fatigue or catarrh. So much for milk's 'body-building' image.

Advertisers are highly paid and skilled at promoting their products, often with the assistance of 'nutritional experts'. The latter are sometimes so careful to 'play it safe', that the information they provide about the effects of food on health can be both mundane and uninspiring. Nutritional information given in educational institutes or in pamphlets in doctors' waiting rooms is no better. And if you take the time to look further yourself into the field of nutrition, you can find yourself burdened under extremely complicated and theoretical textbooks on biochemical pathways and enzyme reactions with nary a mention of 'carrot' or 'bean-sprout'.

A Shift in Emphasis

You are probably sick of the paranoia-breeding attitude expounded by doctors and dentists: 'avoid chocolate/ice cream/butter – or in ten years' time you'll have no teeth/be fat/have a stroke'. Why not take a fresh and uplifting look at foods and see them as possible *health-boosters*? Then choose to eat the ones that will give you an extra 'dice roll' for quick progress in the ultrahealth game. Start by kicking the junk-food habit (perhaps you already have, in which case just skip the next section) and leave behind all those pre-cooked, packaged, ready-in-a-minute 'goodies' complete with the myriad chemicals, food additives, white sugar and refined flour they contain. You'll take a giant step on the ultrahealth board.

Ten Steps to Beat the Energy Breakers
Even with the best will in the world, the Junk-Food Demon can make your transition to ultrahealth quite a challenge. But follow the next ten steps and you'll gradually leave the Junk-Food Demon behind to eat his own cream cakes, chocolate bars and soft drinks. You'll also start to experience the energy and fun of ultra foods.

1. Willpower
The first two barriers to overcome concern attitudes, for instance: 'I've tried to give up junk-foods before – but I just don't have the willpower' and 'I know they're bad for me, but I really do like the taste of the "no-no's".'

If you happen to feel this way your 'willpower' is not innately 'weak', nor is it under the tyrannical control of the Junk-Food Demon. It may surprise you to know that when the old 'should I?/shouldn't I?' conflict arises over a chocolate bar or ice-cream cone it is quite possible that your reason for wanting it is some sort of biochemical upset in your body such as a deficiency in one or other vitamin or mineral, or just a disturbed digestive system. When a body is in real harmony with itself you are usually indifferent to even the most voluptuous chocolate sundae. So forget the battle of the will. Stop blaming yourself and look to strengthening your overall state of health and raising your energy levels instead.

2. The Rewards
Just as the ultrahealth game has an ultimate goal and rewards, so each step along the way will bring little mini-rewards. One of the most important aspects of any change in lifestyle is being aware of the rewards it will bring you and enjoying them as they arrive. What are the junk-free diet bonuses?

- Sparkling eyes and clear glowing skin.
- Strong shiny hair.
- A firm, well-toned body.
- A vanishing pot belly.

- A clear mind.
- A fresh positive outlook on life.

3. Are you a Mars bar?
One of the greatest incentives to rid yourself of junk-foods once and for all is the startling realization that you really are what you eat. By understanding even the most rudimentary biological facts you will see that the food you eat becomes the building blocks of the cells in your body. Take a step back next time you are presented with a plateful of chips, sausages and beans and ask yourself, 'Am I really proud to be a greasy chip?'

4. The Dreadful Cravings
You can't pretend they just don't exist. As Snoopy says, 'It's hard to keep your mind on a diet when your stomach just sent out for a pizza,' so what can you do? First, understand why you have cravings. Many cravings come in the form of a sweet tooth – the feeling that you just must have something sweet – a chocolate bar, some biscuits etc. Then there is the craving for a cup of coffee. As different as they appear, these two are actually linked. They both stem from a need for a boost in energy. You feel a little tired and need pepping up, so you eat chocolate or drink coffee. An hour or two later you find yourself even more tired and with an even stronger craving. And the cycle goes on as you put yet more strain on your pancreas to regulate your blood sugar and deplete your body of yet more of the important vitamins and minerals. Then there are the allergy cravings. You *need* a doughnut or an ice cream – and not just one, but several. Food allergies can leave you feeling ravenously hungry even after eating a large meal. Again, take a step back, and acknowledge your cravings for what they really are – you will not die, nor will you even suffer, without that quick junk-food snack, and the sooner you realize it, the better. Then you can take steps to banish them (see pages 113–14 on food allergies).

5. Substitutes
It's all very well denying yourself this or that, but what do you eat to fill the gap?

- Replace refined grain products with wholemeal ones such as bread, pasta, crackers, noodles and rice.

- Replace ice cream and milk shakes with fresh fruit sorbets, frappés and yogurt lhassis.

- Substitute healthy snick-snacks made by grinding nuts and dried fruit and forming into little balls instead of chocolate bars.

With a little imagination and experimentation you will find that giving up junk-food is no sacrifice at all.

6. Exercise
One of the ways to lose your dependency on junk-food and to do away with cravings is to get plenty of exercise. Exercise will quickly rid your body of metabolic waste products, the presence of which make you crave the junk-food monstrosities. By increasing the amount of oxygen supplied to each cell of your body a regular exercise regime helps cleanse and strengthen your system and finely tune it so that you can no longer stomach junk-foods (see page 49).

7. Drink Like a Fish
Another very helpful way quickly to eliminate toxins from your system is to flush them out by drinking lots of liquids. Spring water is great – it cleanses the digestive tract, liver and kidneys. Unless you practically *live* on a diet of all raw foods, drink at least four glasses a day. Fresh raw vegetable juices are even better for cleaning your cells. Water drinking breeds energy to burn in the body too – as several studies in which athletes were forced to drink large quantities of water show. Herb teas are very useful too. Apart from having their own specific therapeutic properties they are helpful in taking the edge off your appetite when you crave a certain food or feel like a snack (see page 110).

8. Snacks
Probably the time when you are most likely to confront the Junk-Food Demon is when you decide to 'grab a quick bite to eat' to sustain you between meals, or to replace one. If all you can find for a snack is a chocolate bar or packaged apple pie you are better off

going hungry. Missing a snack, or even a meal for that matter, is no terrible sin. On the other hand, if you are hungry, you are hungry. Try to make sure that you have good snacking material at the ready – a piece of fruit or a bag full of crunchy crudités is ideal. Sunflower seeds or unsalted nuts are a good energy sustainer, but make sure they are really fresh and remember they are also high in fat so you may not want to eat them too frequently. One of the bonuses of the ultrahealth way of eating is that you find by eliminating false hunger caused by blood sugar problems, food allergies and cravings, you no longer have the same ravenous appetite between meals.

9. Junk the junk
You can't tell every fast food restaurant to close down or every street vendor to move his cans of fizzy drinks out of your sight, but what you can do is be responsible for the food in your own home. Don't take the attitude that as you bought that large chocolate cake you ought to finish it anyway, and don't let it sit around staring you in the face. Get rid of it, or give it away. The sooner you eliminate 'tempting' foods from your own kitchen, the easier it will be for you to forget about them altogether.

10. Steer Clear of the Traps
Don't let yourself get into difficult situations socially where you are forced to eat bad foods. Anticipate the junk-food traps and be sure to either bring your own foods with you or avoid eating altogether. Don't be afraid to turn down your Aunt Betsy's trifle – you've probably eaten it enough times to convince her that it tastes O.K. and if you show her how determined you are to pursue the ultrahealth way of eating maybe she'll learn to make it (and enjoy it!) with unrefined flour and raw sugar instead. Be determined and don't let obstacles such as cynical remarks from onlookers or 'friends' prevent you from reaching your goal.

These ten points are not only helpful for the 'junk-food addict', but even for people who eat an average 'good' diet. They can help clear the decks for ultrahealth eating. So can ten days on a special spring-cleaning regime – see Chapter Eight.

Sweet Can Be Beautiful
Sugar has received a bad press these last few years, following the

published research of respected nutritionists such as Professor John Yudkin – who labelled it 'pure, white and deadly' – and Professors Ross Hume Hall and Dr Abram Hoffer. All sugars, brown and white, were deemed equally culpable; their alternatives and substitutes – xylitol, glycoside, fructose, saccharine and cyclamates – have never proven themselves really satisfactory. But now that wholesale condemnation has been called into question by recent Russian research.

One of the foremost Russian researchers, Professor I. I. Brekhman of the Far East Scientific Centre of the former USSR Academy of Sciences, elaborates the new thinking in *Brown Sugar and Health*. He and his colleagues have a revisionist attitude to biochemistry, believing that the *quantitative* measure of energy potential contained in foodstuffs – more commonly called calories – is not of the singular importance it was thought to be. Nor does the regular, but generally haphazard, ingestion of foods containing vitamins, minerals, proteins, fats, carbohydrates and fibre, improve one's health noticeably. They believe that not only are certain nutrients, which can be measured chemically, necessary for health but so also is the *way* in which they and other unidentifiable factors combine in individual foods to provide a particular *quality* of energy. This 'way' Brekhman calls 'structural information'. A high degree of structural information enables the food to make the most of its nutrients, to be *biologically active*. In laboratory tests, raw, unrefined sugar has demonstrated a high degree of biological activity comparable to certain other raw foods, including ginseng.

Raw sugar appears to increase resistance to illness, heighten energy levels, and improve an organism's ability to deal with stress. The same has not been shown to be true of white, or even most store-bought 'coloured', sugars. For a sugar to be a 'true' unrefined sugar, it must still contain the thin film of molasses surrounding the sucrose crystal. This contains some 200 organic nutrients which are useful in themselves and are also essential for the breakdown of the sucrose in the body. To recognize the real thing, read the label carefully. Look for the word 'unrefined' and 'golden granulated' and also for the country of origin. If it comes from Barbados, Guyana or Mauritius then you have hit the jackpot; if it is from Malawi or has no country of origin on the label put it back. It will either be of low quality or a white, refined sugar with added colouring. Generally, the darker the colour of the sugar, the higher the proportion of health-protecting elements and structural information it contains.

8
How to Leap Ahead in the Ultrahealth Game

TEN DAYS ON the Biogenic Clean-Up is an excellent way to take a great step towards ultrahealth. It is also a superb method for spring-cleaning – I don't mean carting out boxes of junk from the attic either. I mean detoxifying your body to bring it a new sense of vitality, to regenerate all its systems for maximum good looks and energy. A face and body undergo a remarkable rejuvenation when you spend a fortnight at one of the top European biological clinics. This is almost entirely due to the way these centres use diet and other tools to encourage the rapid elimination of wastes, some of which have been stored in the body for many years. The Biogenic Clean-Up is based on the same principles. It is certainly not *necessary* for achieving ultrahealth, but it can bring you a long way along that path in a hurry if you are keen to make rapid changes for the better.

The human body is magnificently designed to cleanse itself automatically without ever giving thought to the process. The trouble is that the kind of food and drink most people in the west put into it, the tendency we have to lead stressful but sedentary lives, and the increasing number of pollutants to which we are exposed through the air we breathe and the water we drink, have created a situation in which often far more toxins are taken into the body, and far more metabolic wastes are produced in it, than we can effectively get rid of. Instead they are stored in the tissues where they lower vitality, encourage the development of degenerative diseases and early ageing and rob the system of nutrients necessary to keep skin and hair – indeed your whole body – looking their best.

Dr. Dwight McKee, Medical Director of the International

Health Institute in America, put it rather bluntly when he said recently, 'anybody who has lived the mainstream American lifestyle for ten or more years has 70 trillion garbage cans for cells'. McKee believes, as do a growing number of physicians who are using alternative methods for the treatment of cancer and other degenerative illnesses, that our cells are literally chock-full of metabolic and environmental wastes gathered over a lifetime. To live at a high level of health and vitality, not to mention being able to make the most of your potential for good looks and prolonged youth, you need to get rid of them.

Detoxification Begins Here
The Biogenic Clean-Up is designed to spring-clean your body – to begin the process of detoxification and set you on the road to an ultrahealth way of living which is more supportive of high-level vitality and good looks. It is a total programme which involves a temporary change of diet using living foods and eliminating as much as possible those foods which encourage the production of mucoid substances that clog the system. In fact, the programme is structured so that it can do many different things at once, all of them connected with the process of regeneration and renewal, encouraging weight-loss (if you have excess weight to lose), improving the look and texture of your skin and minimizing lines on the face, and re-establishing great biochemical balance in the body, as well as increasing your sense of vitality and wellbeing.

John Douglass MD of the California Permanente Medical Group and other physicians have used such a high-raw diet on diabetics and found that insulin levels can be reduced, and in some cases the need for insulin eliminated altogether. In Switzerland and Germany some of the world's finest clinics use this kind of a biogenic regime. In Britain, a growing number of doctors, discontented with the single-cause theory of illness on which western high-technology medicine is based, are turning towards the kinds of foods used in the Biogenic Clean-Up, not only as a means of treatment for illness but for promoting high energy levels and improving overall wellness.

The Biogenic System
Conventionally, foods are classified into five main groups, and a

well-balanced diet is regarded as one which includes some food from each of the groups. We also tend to measure a food's worth only in terms of calories, protein, fat and carbohydrate content plus the vitamins and minerals it contains. But physicians using the Biogenic Clean-Up for healing approach food differently.

Besides taking into account a food's vitamin and mineral content, they classify foods into four main categories.

Biogenic Foods are those which contain life-generating forces, such as sprouted seeds and sprouted grains, fresh fruit and raw vegetable juices. These foods are used for detoxifying the body, for active healing and rapid biological transformations.

Bioactive Foods – fresh unprocessed whole vegetables and fruits, nuts and raw dairy products – make up the largest part of a Biogenic Clean-Up.

Biostatic Foods, such as cooked vegetables and cooked grains, cooked animal proteins such as fish, meat and game, and shellfish have a natural effect, for they do not usually predispose the body to illness, nor do they contribute much to optimum health. In fact, they tend to slow down bodily processes, so they are used not as the centre of a meal but as a complementary dish, and are not included in any temporary regime for rapid rejuvenation.

Biocidic Foods – tinned, frozen, heavily processed foods, refined and concentrated foods (such as white sugar and white flour), and anything which contains synthetic additives such as chemical preservatives, humectants, emulsifiers, colourings and so on. Since they are considered potentially responsible for the development of disease, they are rigorously avoided. Because the average British or American diet contains a number of biostatic and biocidic foods, it decreases vitality and makes the body more susceptible to early ageing and disease. Its excessive fat and sugar content contributes to the accumulation of wastes in the tissues which impair proper cellular nutrition and encourage the formation of a kind of sludge in the bloodstream that can impede good circulation. Both these things can lead to the formation of cellulite in women and contribute to premature ageing of the skin in both men and women.

The average diet can also burden the body with excessive acidity, which leads to irritability, fatigue, mineral loss and eventually illness. So one of the important aspects of rejuvenation through biogenic foods is simply the removal of a great deal of biological stress, the restoration of the correct acid–alkaline balance, and the elimination of toxic waste products that have been stored in your system. As Max Gerson, who became famous for his cures of serious conditions using biogenic foods, used to say:

> To save the body from extra work in the disposal of excessive foods, especially fats which are difficult to digest, the destruction of poisons etc. is a precaution that may prevent many kinds of early degeneration, premature old age and all kinds of acute and chronic sickness.

The biogenic approach to renewal eliminates all the biocidic foods and all highly processed foods. It also eliminates foods which are the commonest cause of sensitivities, sometimes only temporarily (for with improved nutrition many so-called food allergies disappear), sometimes permanently. The two most common offenders, according to clinical ecologists, who specialize in the identification and treatment of food allergies (see pages 113–14), are cows' milk and wheat. Such physicians claim that sensitivity to these two foods is far more widespread than most people realize and that it can result in the development of a number of common ailments such as arthritis, eczema, constipation, chronic fatigue and many emotional or mental problems such as manic depression. More commonly, people who have an undiagnosed sensitivity to cows' milk and wheat tend to experience a lowering of vitality so that enjoyment of everyday life is far less than it could be. Because this kind of food sensitivity is so common – and because both milk and wheat tend to encourage mucus in the body (more about this later) – the Biogenic Clean-Up eliminates cows' milk and products such as cheese and yogurt which are made from it, and wheat-based products such as bread and pasta, in favour of goats' milk products and breads made from other grains such as rye and oats. (Raw oats, incidentally, are said to contain hormone-like substances which resemble the body's sex hormones and are important for keeping skin smooth and unlined.)

Raw Vitality

As well as their detoxifying properties, the raw seeds, grains, fruits and vegetables which form the basis of biogenic renewal have other remarkable qualities. A German researcher, Tropp Kaspar, showed that, far from being destroyed by digestive processes, the majority of enzymes contained in raw foods are taken through the digestive system to the colon unharmed. There they act on the natural intestinal bacterial flora by attracting and binding any oxygen present. This eliminates the aerobic condition in which harmful bacteria grow and protects the intestines from fermentation, putrefaction and toxaemia – all of which are common problems in the west and which can lead to digestive disturbances and the retention of waste products, interfering with cell metabolism and encouraging rapid ageing.

These natural, health-giving plant enzymes found in raw seeds, grains, fruit and vegetables are destroyed when we cook them. Another European researcher, Werner Kollath, discovered that although a so-called 'normal' state of health could be maintained in animals fed on a diet of cooked foods, they eventually showed signs of degeneration, just as ageing people do. But when he put these animals on a diet of the same foods, *uncooked*, these degenerative changes were avoided. In the early stages many of these changes could even be reversed on raw foods. Kollath concluded that there must be some unknown factors, quite apart from the vitamin and mineral content of raw plant foods, which protect an organism from degeneration and are capable of rejuvenating it as well as healing a large degree of degeneration that has already taken place.

More recent research has shown that certain factors which occur in fresh plant foods but are destroyed by heat, such as the bioflavonoids, abscisic acid and the gibberellins, appear to stimulate the immune system and to help protect the body from illness and age-related changes. Plant hormones known as the secretins may also help to maintain health through a complex kind of feedback control which they can exert through the endocrine system. Other researchers have found that the volatile oils of plant foods favourably affect the digestive system and increase the absorption of nutrients into the bloodstream. All of these benefits from raw foods are combined with the high vitamin and mineral content which is greatly reduced or even destroyed by cooking. Also, cooking at high temperatures can change the essential *cis* fatty acids in foods into harmful *trans* fatty acids which the body cannot make use of.

It is therefore hardly surprising that when healthy people are put on a high-raw diet, as they are in many of the world's fancy spas, most of them look and feel better than ever before. Such a diet is also excellent for active people. Another German professor, Karl Eimer, put top athletes on a raw-food regime, reduced their protein intake from 100 to 50 grammes a day and to his amazement found the men grew stronger, swifter and more supple.

The Biogenic Clean-Up makes use of a lot of living foods – fresh raw vegetables and fruits and sprouted seeds and grains as well as herb teas, spices and (as an option) freshly made vegetable and fruit juices. It also eliminates to a large degree those foods which tend to be mucoid-forming. Just what does this mean?

Beware the Mucoid-Formers

Quite apart from the normal mucus secreted by the body's mucous membranes to keep the linings of the nose and throat and alimentary canal lubricated, the body produces what are often referred to as *mucoids* in response to toxicity or to substances which are potentially harmful to it. Such mucoid matter tends to be thick, slimy and sticky. It is produced in the lungs, in the digestive system, the lymphatics, the reproductive system and even the connective tissues throughout the body. Unlike normal mucus which is transparent and slippery, this excessive mucoid matter tends to be cloudy and thick. What European researchers into the actions of various foods on the body have discovered is that many foods have mucoid-forming properties. These they dubbed *mucoid-forming foods*. This mucoid-producing phenomenon in the digestive system they call 'digestive leucocytosis'. They warn that when people eat a diet which encourages it, as the average western fare does, they not only reduce their resistance to infection but tend to clog their digestive system and lymphatics with stagnant mucoid substances that lower vitality and can encourage the development of chronic illness. Most of the finest natural healing regimes are based on low-mucoid-forming foods. Some people appear to have a particularly high resistance to mucoid-forming influences (which include not only certain foods but pollutants in air, air conditioning and even exposure to some kinds of electronic equipment, apparently because of the action these have on reducing the concentration of negative ions in the air), others have far less. Many researchers believe that the former are probably the people with a very high resistance to illness as well. Some foods are far more inclined to produce mucoids in the body than others. The Biogenic Clean-Up stresses those that are not.

Take a Fresh Look at Food

Dairy products – particularly those made from pasteurized cows' milk – are considered the most mucoid-forming of all foods. Second on the list are the so-called 'high-protein' animal foods such as meat, poultry, fish and eggs. They are included only in the last two 'transition days' of the diet and then only in small quantities. Then come the soya-based foods such as tofu and textured vegetable protein, pulses, nuts and grains in that order. The fruits and vegetables which form the mainstays of the diet are totally non-mucoid-forming. So are sprouted seeds and grains – which are wonderful for lasting good looks and high level vitality. They should become part of your daily diet even after 'spring-cleaning' is finished. For when seeds such as alfalfa, grains such as wheat, and pulses such as chickpeas and mung beans are sprouted, within a few days they lose their mucoid-forming properties completely. They also become nutritional powerhouses – rich in vitamins and minerals, essential amino acids and easy to digest natural sugars. And they are delicious as the basis of the most exquisite raw vegetable salads which make great meals in themselves. You can buy ready-sprouted seeds from healthfood shops and supermarkets or, better, purchase seeds such as: alfalfa, mung beans, aduki beans, lentils, chickpeas and wheat from healthfood shops or seed suppliers and sprout your own.

Making Your Own Yogurt

From really fresh goats' milk you can make yogurt without scalding the milk simply by adding a culture and raising the temperature to lukewarm. Bought goats' milk can be scalded, then cooled to lukewarm before adding the culture and placing in a commercial yogurt maker or an earthenware pot or large jar in a warm place for eight to ten hours. Then refrigerate. A tablespoon of ordinary plain yogurt will do fine for a 'start' culture to a pint of goats' milk. Save a tablespoon or two from each batch of yogurt to start the next batch with.

Goats' Milk Yogurt

Goats' milk is one of the most nutritious sources of raw protein, used by Hippocrates for healing in Greek times. It is much finer and more digestible than cows' milk, with smaller fat globules, and is richer in the simple fatty acids. It is also naturally homogenized, and has a mild laxative effect. Because of its higher phosphate content it is of great value in vegetarian or semi-vegetarian diets. It also has a higher vitamin B1 content than cows' milk and is wonderful for anyone who suffers from sensitivity or allergy to cows' milk, or skin troubles (it is often used to treat eczema).

A delicious soft goats' cheese can be made by putting goats' yogurt into a muslin bag and letting it drain for an hour or two. You can then add chopped herbs or garlic or spices to season it.

Getting Down to Business

The Biogenic Clean-Up is in three parts. The first part – two days – is a highly alkaline regime which works best if you can use raw fruit and vegetable juices made in a centrifuge juice extractor; otherwise they can be bought from healthfood stores. The German firm Biotta make some juices bottled at very low temperatures to preserve their enzyme, vitamin and mineral content, and Aspell apple juice is also bottled in this way. These help to accelerate the elimination of accumulated toxins and wastes and restore a good potassium balance. The second part – six days – is designed to introduce you to the biogenic way of eating and give you some experience of how different it can make you feel while the raw foods go to work rebalancing, rebuilding and revitalizing your system. The final two days are designed as prototypes for a long-term way of eating that keeps you looking young and feeling superb.

Do-It-Yourself Sprouting

Take a jam jar and put a handful of seeds into it – mung, alfalfa, lentils, fenugreek, for instance. Fill it with bottled water and let it sit for eight hours or overnight with a piece of cheesecloth or nylon stocking secured over the top of it. Then pour off all the water through the cloth top and fill it with fresh water, rinsing the seeds a couple of times through the cloth. Now turn the jar upside down so it drains away any excess water, and leave it to sit.

Repeat this kind of watering and draining twice a day and by the third to the fifth day you will have perfectly delicious fresh sprouts to make salads with. Refrigerate any you don't use right away – they will keep for at least a week.

(It is a good idea, on the Biogenic Clean-Up, to start your sprouts on the pre-diet day or even before so that they are ready on day four when you need them.)

When seeds, grains and pulses are sprouted in this way their vitamin content increases up to 700 per cent. This includes vitamins A, B complex, C, E, and K – even vitamin B12, which is hard to find in vegetables.

Stocking the Kitchen
There are a few foods in the Biogenic Clean-Up which may be new to you, such as goats' milk yogurt, the 'three seeds', and herb teas. They can be found in healthfood stores and the recipes in this chapter.

The Wonderful 'Three Seeds'
The diet also calls for the 'three-seed mixture' – equal parts of sunflower seeds, sesame seeds and pumpkin seeds chopped finely in a food processor, blender or coffee grinder. They should be freshly ground and sprinkled on salads. They are a good source of essential fatty acids and encourage the production of important enzymes. Mixed together they are also an excellent complete protein. Sunflower seeds themselves boast outstanding nutritive properties. One of the world experts in using diet to cure disease and to promote high-level health, Dr. John Douglass, discovered that raw sunflower seeds, together with a few green leaves which contain vitamin C and vitamin A, are also capable of supporting life and health. He points out that they are a good source of B complex vitamins, protein and calories and that, pound-for-pound, they contain 25 times more thiamine than steak, three and a half times as much iron, twice the protein and a good quantity of vitamin E.

Drinks
Throughout the diet you may drink lots of spring water or herb teas

liberally between meals. (For herb teas and beverages see pages 106–110.) Season all your food with fresh herbs, mustard, pepper, cayenne and spices – not with salt, which can upset the potassium–sodium balance of your body and encourages water retention, and possibly more serious problems. Of course you can also use a vegetable broth powder without additives in salad dressings, soups and main dishes.

The Biogenic Clean-Up
This diet is designed for healthy people. It does not claim to be curative. As with any dramatic change in regime, it is wise to check with your physician before embarking on it.

Elimination: **Days 1 and 2**

FIRST THING: A cup (hot or cold) of spring water with the juice of half a lemon and a little honey if desired.

BREAKFAST: A large glass of fresh raw fruit juice (apple, orange, grape, grapefruit, etc.), freshly squeezed. You can drink as much as you like since there are no restrictions on amounts of raw juices and vegetables. Herb tea, with honey if desired.

A piece of fruit in season, a bunch of black grapes or a bowl of cherries.

LUNCH: A large glass or two of fresh raw vegetable juice; choose any mixture you like of carrots, raw beetroot, celery, cucumber, cabbage, tomato, spinach, etc. Carrot juice has a pleasant sweet taste and is a good base for any juice mixture to which small amounts of other vegetables can be added. Almond tonic (see recipe, page 94).

DINNER: Same as breakfast.

THROUGHOUT THE DAY: Drink as much water or herb tea, sweetened with honey if desired (see pages 106, 110 for suggestions), or natural spring water (Perrier, Badoit, Vittel, Volvic or Evian) as you like.

Rebalancing: **Days 3, 4, 5, 6, 7, 8**

FIRST THING: A cup of lemon and spring water *or* herb tea.

BREAKFAST: Fruit, fresh juice *or* a raw breakfast dish *or* drink (see recipes).

LUNCH: A large glass of fresh raw vegetable juice sprinkled with fresh herbs and seasoned with a teaspoon of lemon juice. A large biogenic salad (see recipes) sprinkled with three-seed mixture, *or* goats' cheese, *or* mixed nuts (hazelnuts, almonds, walnuts etc.). A piece of fruit *or* Banana Treat.

DINNER: A large glass of fresh vegetable juice *or* a chilled raw soup (see recipes). A raw main dish (see recipes) with a small side salad *or* a large salad as at lunch.
Fruit *or* muesli (see recipes).
Herb tea *or* coffee substitute such as Pioneer, Barley Cup or Dandelion Coffee.

Long-term Prototype: **Days 9 and 10**

FIRST THING: A cup of herb tea *or* lemon and spring water.

BREAKFAST: Fresh raw fruits in season *or* fresh raw fruit juice. A raw breakfast dish *or* drink (see recipes). A piece or two of 100% rye *or* pumpernickel bread *or* toast with honey.
Herb tea *or* coffee substitute.

LUNCH: Crudités, avocado vinaigrette *or* a glass of fresh vegetable juice.
A biogenic salad (see below).
A slice of rye crispbread with herb goats' cheese if desired. Fruit, yogurt *or* muesli.
Herb tea *or* coffee substitute.

DINNER: Fresh vegetable juice *or* raw soup *or* crudités.
A raw main dish *or* grilled fish, *or* lamb's liver *or* free-range chicken, *or* game. A jacket potato *or* brown rice *or* rye *or* pumpernickel bread.

A small salad *or* lightly cooked fresh vegetables.
A piece of fruit *or* sorbet.
Herb tea *or* coffee substitute.
(Lunch and dinner can be swapped round.)

The Biogenic Recipe Rota
Raw breakfast dishes and drinks

BLACK MAGIC
1 glass goats' milk
1 ripe banana
1–2 tbsp blackstrap molasses (unsulphured)
Blend and serve.

FRUIT SHAKE
1 banana (or peach, or 2 apricots, or figs or berries)
1 glass fresh orange, apple or mandarin juice
1 raw egg yolk
ice cubes
Blend and serve.

LIVE MUESLI
1–2 tbsp breakfast oats, soaked overnight in a little spring water
1 grated apple (or mango, peach, strawberries)
goats' milk yogurt
Mix all ingredients and sprinkle with three-seed mixture or mixed
nuts.

RAW BREAKFAST CEREAL
2 tbsp wheatgerm
2 tbsp three-seed mixture
1 sliced banana or other fruit
1 tsp honey
1 tbsp lecithin
Mix and serve with goats' milk.

CAROB LHASSI
1 glass goats' milk
1 tsp lecithin

1 tbsp three-seed mixture
1 tsp carob powder
1 tbsp honey
Blend and serve.

ALMOND TONIC
15 fresh almonds
1 tsp honey
Blanch almonds, remove the skins, then liquidize with honey and a
large glass of spring water.

Biogenic salads

The principles of biogenic salad-making are simple. Mix together
no more than three vegetables – one root, one bulb (or 'fruit')
vegetable, and one leaf vegetable. Garnish with fresh or dried herbs
and add dressing.

Root vegetables: carrots, celeriac, turnips, onions, leeks, beetroot,
radishes, white radishes etc.

Bulb or 'fruit' vegetables: tomatoes, red and green peppers, fennel,
avocado, cucumber, cauliflower, celery, broccoli, courgettes,
mushrooms, calabrese, etc.

Leaf vegetables: lettuce, young dandelion leaves, young beet tops, red
or white cabbage, Brussels sprouts, spring greens, spinach, chicory,
endive, etc. Watercress, cress and sprouted grains and seeds can be
used in any combination or on their own or as a garnish.

To increase a salad's protein content you can sprinkle it with the
three-seed mixture, or mixed nuts or sprouted seeds or grains, or
add some soft goats' cheese.

SPROUT SALAD
Mix three kinds of sprouted grains or seeds (a handful of each) in a
bowl, add half a sliced avocado and season with fresh basil and
chives. Garnish with black olives and dress with garlic dressing.

SPINACH SPLENDOUR
2 cups spinach
1 cup fresh mushrooms
Remove stems and veins of spinach. Slice mushrooms finely and mix together. Toss in garlic dressing and sprinkle with basil, sunflower seeds or three-seed mixture.

RED SLAW
1½ cups grated cabbage
1 grated carrot
½ grated green pepper
1 tbsp honey
a pinch of celery seeds
Toss with salad dressing and serve.

SALAD DRESSING
Mix one part lemon juice and two parts fresh unrefined cold pressed olive oil or four parts mashed avocado. Add herbs, garlic, mustard or honey to this base.

Raw main dishes

STUFFED LETTUCE
iceberg lettuce leaves
2 tbsp soft goats' cheese
1 small carrot, grated finely
2 tsp fresh chopped herbs
a tiny piece of crushed garlic if desired
Mix the ingredients together then roll up inside the crisp lettuce leaves and serve.

PÂTÉ VIVANTE
1 grated medium carrot
1 chopped spring onion
1 tbsp chopped celery
1 tsp chopped mushrooms
1 tsp lemon juice
1 raw egg yolk
2 tbsp three-seed mixture (or mixed nuts)
Mix together and form into patties.

Raw Soups

CUCUMBER
1 cup goats' milk yogurt
1/2 cucumber, peeled and sliced
sprig of mint
1 tsp lemon juice
Blend and serve sprinkled with parsley.

GAZPACHO
4–6 peeled tomatoes
3 carrots
2 sticks of celery
a dash of cayenne
Put through a centrifuge juicer, sprinkle with chopped chives and diced green pepper.

AVOCADO SMOOTHIE
3/4 cup goats' milk yogurt
1/2 avocado
1/4 diced red pepper
1 tsp lemon juice
1 chopped spring onion
a dash of Tabasco
Blend and serve.

9
Eating for Ultrahealth

WHETHER OR NOT you use the Biogenic Clean-Up to advance quickly in the ultrahealth game, or decide to take a slower, steadier approach, the principles outlined in it form the basis of the entire ultrahealth way of nutrition – a way in which you eat plenty of *biogenic* and *bioactive* foods, very few *biostatic* foods and eliminate completely the *biocidic* foods. In this way you focus on the foods that will bring you positive health benefits and high energy. As in the Biogenic Clean-Up, fuel for the ultrahealth way of eating comes primarily from fruits and vegetables – many of them eaten raw and from wholegrains, pulses and seeds (best if they are sprouted) – plus small quantities of fish and game if you like, and a very little meat if you absolutely *must* – but flesh foods are entirely optional. It is a way of eating which is low in fat, moderate in protein compared to the average western fare – and eliminates completely refined carbo-hydrates and sugars, as well as all highly-processed packaged foods. Here is a brief outline of the ultrahealth nutritional principles:

A Drastic Change From What You're Used To?
For some the ultrahealth approach to nutrition will seem a very different way of eating from what they are used to – eliminating the sweets, white flour and large quantities of meat and gravy. For instance, if you are used to putting lots of butter on your foods, it seems strange at first to eat so little of it. But it is fairly simple to learn to cook foods without lots of fats and oils and to eat them without adding salt, to eliminate the sugary foods and the things made from white flour and to get used to all the pulses and grains and the sparseness of animal protein which the diet calls for.

Whether you embrace the entire ultrahealth way of eating or simply adjust your usual way of eating to bring it more in line with the dietetic principles (no sugar, low fat, low animal protein and no extra salt), within only a few weeks you will find that you are on to something good to make you look younger, feel better than ever before and maybe even live longer.

An Ultrahealth Menu

ON RISING: A cup of hot water to which the juice of half a lemon has been added, to help alkalinize your system and to promote complete elimination.

BREAKFAST: Half a grapefruit, a mango, some cherries or other fresh fruit.
A bowl of Live Muesli (see page 93) *or* a bowl of wholegrain porridge with a sliced banana, skimmed milk, a dash of cinnamon and a tablespoon of honey.

LUNCH: A large mixed salad of raw vegetables dressed with a light dressing made from yogurt or lemon juice or olive oil and cider vinegar and sprinkled with chopped eggs, sunflower seeds, low-fat cheese or minced chopped nuts. Wholegrain toast if desired.

DINNER: A fresh raw salad of tomato, cucumber and watercress, tossed with plenty of sprouts.
4 oz grilled chicken from which the skin has been removed.
A selection of fresh vegetables such as cauliflower, broccoli or courgettes steamed or wok-fried and served with fresh or dried herbs and spices instead of butter and salt, or added raw to your salad.
A piece of wholemeal Greek pitta bread or a portion of long-grain brown rice, or a baked potato.
Fresh strawberries.

For snacks you can eat fresh fruit, wholewheat rolls stuffed with salad, pitta bread, raw sunflower seeds.

The Ultrahealth Fat-Loss Bonus

One of the particularly appealing aspects of the ultrahealth regime is that eating in this way, most people find they reduce any excess fat slowly and steadily without ever having to count calories. This is because the ultrahealth way of eating eliminates excess fats from the diet and is rich in natural fibre from fresh raw vegetables, whole grains and pulses. Fat offers more calories per ounce than any other food. A mere tablespoon of olive oil contains 125 calories – about three or four times what you'll find in a large salad – minus the dressing. You can actually get used to doing without butter on everything and substituting light yogurt-based dressings for oil and vinegar on some of your salads. With the ultrahealth way of eating you still get about 20 to 25 per cent of your total calories in fat, for even the foods themselves contain fat. Indeed, people who have been on such a low-fat diet for several months show no signs of the excessively dry skin which would indicate a fat deficiency.

But there are other reasons why the ultrahealth diet is useful for shedding fat. Because it is mostly made up of complex carbo-hydrates which – unlike sugar and products made from refined flour – are only slowly metabolized, the diet is able to supply a slow and steady stream of energy to the body throughout the day. This keeps you from being hungry and prevents the drastic alterations in blood-sugar levels which lead to fatigue and hunger.

Shopping for Ultrahealth Foods

The shelves of our supermarkets and the tables in our best restaurants are full of delicious foods and dishes which do little to promote ultrahealth but which use up a great deal of the precious adaptive energy you need to help you deal with stress, stay young-looking and ward off illness. Often they are made from refined flour and contain food additives and preservatives. The typical packaged, ready-in-a-minute meal tends to be high in 'hidden' fats, and often sugars too. All these things – excess fats, sugar, refined carbo-hydrates and food additives – put your body under stress and don't belong in an ultrahealth lifestyle . . . So what does?

'Virtuous' Vegetables

What's so special about vegetables? Plenty. They have powerful protective properties, which is why diets high in fresh vegetables are currently being recommended as an aid to protecting the body from degenerative diseases such as cancer, arthritis and arteriosclerosis. Even more important to the ultrahealth player, a diet high in *raw* vegetables will actually increase the microelectric potentials of your body's tissues, making cells function better, improving inter- and extra-cellular exchange and imparting high levels of mental and physical vitality to your whole being. An increasing number of studies are also beginning to show that certain vegetables contain specific plant factors which can greatly enhance health. Fresh vegetables are a rich source of natural fibre, vitamins and minerals for high-level wellness.

Cabbage vs Cancer

Vegetables in the cabbage family, including cauliflower, broccoli, turnips and Brussels sprouts – contain natural carcinogen inhibitors known as *indoles*. Studies have shown that a large percentage of animals who are administered cancer-causing chemicals but at the same time given these foods will not develop cancer. Even human studies show that people who eat the most cabbage are least likely to develop cancer of the colon. Cabbage also contains selenium, a substance found in many plants, which boosts the action of vitamin E in the body. Selenium has been related statistically to low-incidence cancer rates while vitamin E is believed to be another natural carcinogen-inhibitor.

But the cabbages are by no means the only vegetables with the capacity to help prevent degenerative diseases. At the world's most famous biological clinics, such as the Bircher-Benner hospital in Zürich, a diet high in an assortment of fresh raw vegetables has proven effective in the treatment of many different illnesses, from cancer and arthritis to circulatory ailments, diabetes and even many mental disorders. One possible explanation is that, due to their high fibre content, raw vegetables have the ability to speed up the digestive process and decrease the overall time it takes for food to pass through you. This is of particular importance in the case of cancer of the colon for it means that there is less time for intestinal bacteria to convert bile acids into carcinogenic compounds. Lack of bulk in most people's diets is directly related to high incidence of degenerative diseases.

Special Information for Disease-Avoiders
Why is ultrahealth eating so different from the average western fare? Because to produce high-level vitality, protection from degeneration and illness and combat ageing it *has* to be. A large number of epidemiological studies show that the modern western diet is responsible to a great degree for our illnesses. Many dietary studies have now produced evidence linking our excessive intake of fats, cholesterol and refined carbohydrates, such as sugar and white flour, with the development of degenerative diseases. Researchers such as Nathan Pritikin, who founded the Pritikin Longevity Center in America, and Dean Ornish MD, have been able to show that by changing such a diet – eliminating the apparent 'trouble-makers' – such as fat, sugar and refined carbohydrates – the health of the suffering person can be significantly improved. By implication, if through improved nutrition you can largely avoid the suffering caused by arteriosclerosis, hypertension and other dangerous conditions, you should also be able to use diet as 'preventative medicine' in order to increase lifespan and improve the quality of your life.

In the west 40 to 50 per cent of our daily calories come from fats. This includes not just the obvious fat on meat but the fat contained in milk and cheese, butter, margarine and cooking oil plus the many 'hidden fats' in frozen, convenience foods, breads and cakes. In the primitive societies of developing countries, where people live on a diet of mostly unrefined carbohydrates, little or no sugar and very little fat, our common illnesses, from varicose veins and coronary heart disease to diverticular disease, are virtually unknown. That is, until a typical western diet, including white bread, sugary foods and so on, arrives. Then these illnesses begin rapidly to appear.

Why a Change of Diet Tactics is in Order
The ultrahealth way of eating may be not only radically different from what you are used to, but may seem to overthrow many of the standard established nutritional beliefs about 'meat and two veg'. For instance, you have probably been told that a high protein diet which relies heavily on meat and fish is best to keep you well and strong.

The High-Protein Fallacy

The need for protein has been grossly exaggerated and most of us in the west get far more than we need. Contrary to popular opinion, too much protein can be harmful. Yes, your body needs the constituents of protein – amino acids – for its metabolic processes: growth, the repair and maintenance of bodily tissue and the production of hormones and enzymes. But when it gets more protein than it needs through your diet, the body is forced to shed precious minerals and trace elements such as zinc, calcium, magnesium, iron and chromium. All these nutrients are vital – not only to health and the maintenance of firm skin and shining hair, but to your emotional wellbeing. There is also evidence that a high-protein diet – especially a diet high in meat – plays a leading role in the genesis of osteoporosis and raises the uric acid level which can lead to gout. Finally (again contrary to popular belief) too much protein can also encourage the development of blood sugar problems.

The Meat Myth

The idea that you need to eat meat to stay healthy is also untrue; a mixed diet of roots, grains, vegetables and fruits – all in minimally processed form – is a much better source of higher quality protein than the traditional meat, fish and dairy products which are often very high in fat and too concentrated. Eat meat, fish and game by all means if you want, but only in small quantities – no more than one and a half pounds of flesh foods a week (about three and a half ounces a day) and make sure it is *really* lean. Even the leanest cut of steak boasts over 50 per cent of its calories from fat. Remember too that the vegetables you eat also contain a good quantity of protein, as do pulses – particularly when they are eaten together with grains. Thus a bowl of chili beans eaten together with a piece of wholegrain bread will give you the full complement of the essential amino acids. You need not eat flesh foods at all. And, only 15 to 20 per cent of your daily calories should come from protein-rich food.

Why Stress *Unrefined* Carbohydrates?

Another common assumption which the ultrahealth way of eating challenges is the idea that you mustn't eat too many carbohydrates because 'starches are not really good for you'. In fact carbohydrates are excellent foods for ultrahealth, provided, of course, they are the right kind of carbohydrates, that is *complex* carbohydrates: unrefined grains, pulses, vegetables and fruits eaten in as natural a state as possible. Small quantities of starches such as brown rice or wheat, oats, barley and rye (which have not been milled to death and deprived of most of their natural vitamins, minerals and fibre), when taken together with fresh, preferably raw, vegetables, provide a steady stream of energy which, unlike that from sugar and over-refined starchy foods made from white flour, will never over-stimulate the pancreas and encourage the development of unstable blood sugar levels, obesity or diabetes.

Leaping the Fat Hurdle

There is nothing wrong with fats – in small quantities. In fact, essential fatty acids – linoleic and linolenic acids – are necessary for growth, and for healthy blood, arteries and nerves. They also help keep your skin young by preventing dryness. They appear to be necessary for the transport and breakdown of cholesterol – an important constituent of much body tissue, particularly the nerves, brain, blood and liver. But you need these essential fatty acids only in *very small* quantities. When any kind of fats are taken in greater amounts than your body requires they can act in extremely destructive ways. Excessive fats raise cholesterol and uric acid levels in the tissues. This contributes to gout and arteriosclerosis. They also interfere with proper metabolism of carbohydrates and therefore encourage the development of diabetes. And they create a situation in which your body's cells are deprived of the oxygen they need to function efficiently – a condition known as 'tissue anoxia'. In many ways this tendency of fats to deprive body tissues of the oxygen they need appears to be most serious of all the implications of taking in excess fat. Tissue anoxia is a basic feature of many degenerative diseases – from angina and the development of malignancies to premature ageing. Fats can also hinder our immune system by inhibiting the antibody response as well as the actions of leucocytes – white blood cells which ingest and kill bacteria. And it is not only saturated animal fats that you have to be wary of. New evidence indicates that large quantities of polyunsaturated vegetable oils such as corn oil, safflower oil and sunflower oil can be just as harmful to health. Dr. Kenneth Carroll, a biochemist at the University of Ontario, showed that animals fed exclusively on unsaturated fats developed twice as many tumours as those fed on saturated meat and butter fats.

Too Much Fat Dulls the Brain

Experiments have shown that when someone eats a meal high in *any* kind of fat, the fats form a film round the red blood cells and platelets and encourages them to stick together or clump. This clumping causes small capillaries to clog and even shut down so that as much as 20 per cent of your normal blood circulation is lost, reducing the amount of oxygen available to your cells by about 30 per cent. This clumping and its corresponding oxygen-cell deficit lasts for many hours after eating a meal high in fat. The action of fat on the brain is one of the main reasons why you can feel sleepy or unable to think clearly after eating a heavy meal. Too much fat in your diet interferes with the high-level awareness and mental clarity that goes with ultrahealth. Particularly dangerous are processed unsaturated fats found in cooking oils, margarines and convenience foods.

Hit Out Against Sugar

Sugar also comes under the ultrahealth axe. By now it is common knowledge that the consumption of refined sugar is linked with the development of degenerative illnesses. Sugar, the end of a complex refining process which takes away every vitamin, mineral and trace of natural fibre from the beets or cane from which it is made, is a food virtually empty of nutritional benefit – except for the calories it supplies. Eating sugar tends to raise the level of your blood fats and to put stress on your pancreas, challenging it to maintain normal blood sugar levels. Sugar can also contribute to the development of arteriosclerosis. Yet most of us eat about two pounds a week of the stuff. In fact, about 20 to 25 per cent of our daily calories come from it. The ultrahealth way of eating eliminates refined sugar and all things made from it.

Scrap the Salt

The average western diet contains far too much salt, which causes oedema and also tends to deprive your body's tissues of oxygen. Salt is the major contributor to chronic high blood pressure as well. It also contributes to a great variety of circulatory problems including arthritis, reduced auditory, visual and tactile sensations and causes much muscle and joint stiffness.

Coffee, the 'Pick-me-up-throw-me-down' Drink

Coffee drinking leads to chronic fatigue. Caffeine, like concentrated sugar, stimulates the pancreas to produce more insulin. If you regularly drink a lot of coffee your pancreas can become 'trigger-happy' so that too much insulin is produced, thus lowering the blood sugar levels. This can result in hypoglycaemia and the chronic fatigue that accompanies it, which, in a kind of vicious circle, leads to more coffee drinking.

One of the best things you can give up to improve your skills in the ultrahealth game is coffee. Just a few cups a day of this supposedly innocuous drink can both undermine your wellbeing and help you to age long before your time. Coffee contains caffeine and caffeine is a drug. One of the xanthine groups of chemicals, it stimulates the central nervous system, pancreas and heart as well as the cerebral cortex – which is why, when you drink it, you feel temporarily more alert. It also acts as a mild diuretic and relaxes the smooth muscles such as the bronchials. Every time you drink a cup of coffee you are getting between 90 and 120 mg of caffeine. (A cup of ordinary tea yields 40 to 100 mg, cocoa or cola drinks 20 to 50 mg). If you drink two to eight cups of coffee a day, you are getting a dose of the drug which any pharmacologist would reckon considerable. Taken day after day such a dose can be dangerous.

Caffeine has been shown to affect the heart, causing it to beat rapidly and irregularly. It can also increase the level of free fatty acids in your blood, stimulate the secretion of excess acid in the stomach and raise blood pressure. This raised blood lipid level is one of the suspected factors in arteriosclerosis, while secretion of excess acid in the stomach makes people 1.4 times more susceptible to gastric ulcers. Recent studies have also linked habitual coffee drinking to certain mental illnesses – from quite simple depression and anxiety neurosis to overt psychosis. Caffeine, like the amphetamines which go into 'diet pills', can set off psychotic behaviour by acting on neurotransmitters – chemicals in your brain which carry information across the tiny synapses between the nerve cells. The phenomenon of caffeine producing mental and emotional aberrations is termed 'caffeinism'.

Are You a Caffeine Addict?
Also interesting is caffeine's effect on the body when you stop drinking coffee. For coffee, if you are a steady 'user', is addictive. Its removal can cause powerful withdrawal symptoms. These usually appear as a nausea or headache lasting from a few hours to several days, depending on how serious the addiction and how finely tuned your system is. But the withdrawal symptoms are short-lived and worth going through to be rid of caffeine once and for all.

Ultrahealth Alternative Beverages
Do not fear that the list of 'what not to eat' is going to severely limit the variety of foods and drinks in your diet to the point of subsisting on celery sticks and water (spring water at that!), because for every item on the 'don't' list there is an alternative 'do' with positive health benefits.

So what do you drink instead of tea and coffee?

Coffee Substitutes
The best coffee substitutes usually don't resemble coffee very much in anything but colour, but nevertheless they can be delicious in their own right. They are usually made from chicory and barley or dandelion root, together with spices, and are good sweetened with a little honey and made with hot milk or hot water topped with milk. Good varieties include Dandelion Coffee, Pioneer and Barley Cup. Hot goats' milk with honey and cinnamon, or with a little carob powder and honey, makes a nice replacement for cocoa. Another good hot drink can be made by adding hot water to a pure concentrated fruit juice such as apple or blackcurrant which can be found in healthfood shops.

Ultrahealth Makers and Breakers
No matter how 'well-balanced' your diet is, certain foods, from the word go, are going to boost you towards your ultrahealth goal while others are going to set you back. Of the positive foods some are exceptionally well-endowed with health-promoting goodies – vitamins, minerals, enzymes etc. I call these the 'Health Makers'.

Take brewer's yeast, for example: a protein food, yeast is one of the best sources of B complex vitamins available. It has a mere 25 calories per teaspoon and is rich in nucleic acids – a useful ingredient in encouraging cell renewal. Seaweed – or kelp – offers perhaps the most abundant natural supply of minerals available, containing over 20 different kinds of minerals, including many difficult-to-find, but important, trace minerals. Its high iodine content helps to improve the functioning of the thyroid gland which can promote weight-loss. Seaweed is even said to be useful in combating the ill effects of radiation on the body.

Then there are the 'Health Breakers'. These will not only be of no use but are likely to be a handicap and prevent you from reaching your ultrahealth goal. They are best eliminated from your diet altogether.

The Health Makers

- Sprouted seeds and grains
- Fresh vegetable juices
- Natural unsweetened yogurt – especially goats' milk yogurt
- Fermented foods – natural sauerkraut (for instance)
- Liver
- Molasses
- Wheatgerm
- Pulses and legumes
- Brewer's yeast
- Wholegrains
- Seaweed
- Fresh vegetables

The Health Breakers

- Refined sugar and flour and products made from them
- Preservatives, additives
- Artificial flavouring, colouring, stabilizers, emulsifiers, etc.
- Alcohol, coffee
- Processed fats such as margarines
- Excess fat, excess protein
- Processed foods containing junk-foods

- In fact, anything in excess. Overeating is one of the worst health breakers of all

What about Supplementary Vitamins and Minerals?

Controversy rages over whether or not you need to take supplementary vitamins and minerals if you are following a good dietary lifestyle such as the ultrahealth one. If you do not live in a city and you eat most of your foods out of your own garden, where they have been organically grown, you probably don't. If not, most experts in nutrition and health insist it is a wise thing to do. But how do you choose a formula? By carefully reading labels and by knowing what you are looking for. Basically there are two ways to go when it comes to food supplements – the conservative 'guard against any possible deficiencies', and the more avant-garde mega nutrient approach which is based on the notion that nutritional supplements should be used to counter pollution, protect against ageing and the belief that in larger quantities they may be able to increase energy levels and promote an even higher level of health. If you decide to take supplements you will probably find the ones you choose will lie somewhere between the two extremes. If you like the idea of lower potency supplements with high bio-availability, you might consider food-state vitamins. These are vitamins which have been bonded to food proteins to render them highly bio-available. This means that you can take them in lower doses. The conservative approach is the column on the left, the mega nutrient approach you will find in the right-hand column. This is only offered as a general guide. In no way is it meant to be prescriptive. Ideally you should consult a well-trained nutritionist or doctor who is knowledgeable about supplements to work out an ideal programme for you.

Supplements	Conservative approach	Mega approach
Vitamin A	5,000 IU	25,000 IU
Betacarotene or mixed Carotenoids	15 mg	30–45 mg
Vitamin B1	25 mg	50–100 mg
Vitamin B2	25 mg	50–100 mg
Vitamin B3	25 mg	30–100 mg

Pantothenic Acid	25 mg	50–200 mg
Vitamin B6	10 mg	50–100 mg
Vitamin B12	40 mcg	100 mcg
Folic Acid	200 mcg	800–4,000 mcg
Biotin	100 mcg	300–5,000 mcg
Choline	50 mg	75–500 mg
Inositol	50 mg	75–500 mg
PABA	50 mg	100 mg
Vitamin C	500 mg	2,000–12,000 mg
Bioflavonoids	50 mg	100–500 mg
Vitamin D	300 IU	400 IU
Vitamin E	100 IU	200–2,000 IU
Calcium	100 mg	400–1,600 mg
Magnesium (best as chelated)	50 mg	250–1,000 mg
Potassium	10 mg	50–200 mg
Iron	10 mg	25 mg
Copper	0.5 mg	3 mg
Zinc (best as citrate or picolinate)	10 mg	15–40 mg
Manganese	2 mg	5 mg
Molybdenum	50 mcg	75 mcg
Chromium (best as GTF or pico-linate)	25 mcg	75 mcg
Selenium (best as selenomethionine)	100 mcg	200–400 mcg
Iodine	50 mcg	75–200 mcg
Boron	1 mcg	2 mcg

(If you have any trouble with digestion, digestive enzymes may be required.)

There is one final aspect for an ultrahealth player to consider about foods: how specific foods can affect your mind and body for better or worse because of possible food sensitivities or simply because of the specific effects of the foods themselves. This is a part of nutrition which is seldom considered. Knowing a bit about it cannot only help you avoid such troubles as chronic fatigue and mood swings, it can also help you use food for relaxation, for stimulating energy and for a number of other helpful purposes.

Herb Teas

You can make a wonderful refreshing cup of herb tea using single herbs or herbs and spices in combination. Herb combinations can be found in healthfood shops – loose or in sachets. Some of the most delicious single teas include:

- **Peppermint**
  great for settling an upset stomach
- **Lemon Verbena or Lemon Grass**
  both good tonics
- **Camomile**
  calms the nerves
- **Golden Rod (Solidago)**
  a good diuretic for those who retain water
- **Lime Blossom or Passion Flower**
  good for relaxing you

TIPS

The trick to making good cups of herb tea is first to find several herbs or herb combinations which you enjoy and then to add one or several of the following:

- a squeeze of lemon juice or a slice of lemon

- a teaspoon or so of lightly scented clear honey such as acacia or clover

- a drop of goats' milk or skimmed milk (especially nice with spicy teas)

- a dash of powdered cinnamon bark stick

- Try making a strong pot of your favourite tea and adding a sliced peach to it. Sweeten with honey, then chill for a couple of hours in the fridge and drink iced in tall glasses.

	What to Eat	**What not to Eat**
Meat, Fish, Game and Poultry	Chicken and turkey preferably without the skin which is too fat. Very lean free-range organic fish, game, meat or offal cooked without fat (no more than 4 oz a day).	Ham, sausages, bacon, smoked meats, salmon, tinned tuna. Fatty beef, lamb & pork.
Grains, Breads and Cereals	All wholegrains such as brown rice, millet, wholewheat, rolled oats, breads, wholewheat pasta, pitta bread, Essene bread, crispbreads.	Bread or pastry products made with sugar or bleached white flour, white biscuits and scones.
Pulses	All beans, peas and lentils.	
Fats and Oils	Very little, except what occurs naturally in the grains, seeds, nuts, vegetables and fruits, only small amounts of butter and cold-pressed virgin olive oil (a monosaturated oil).	Margarine, fat on meats and in poultry skins. Processed golden oils and foods containing them, fried foods.
Fruits and Vegetables	All fruits (but no more than five portions a day), all vegetables (unlimited amounts) eaten raw, steamed or lightly cooked in a little soy or olive oil in a wok or baked and cooked without fat.	

Dairy Products	Goats' milk, low-fat cheeses and yogurt (up to 8 oz a day). Cheese made from skimmed milk, yogurt made from skimmed milk (2 oz a day).	Whole milk and cream, most cheeses (too fat and chemically fermented), tinned milk.
Sweets, Drinks and Spices	Fresh fruit, decaffeinated coffee, herb teas, vinegar, fresh or dried herbs, spices, cayenne pepper.	Coffee, tea, sugar, sugared drinks, sugar-free soft drinks, chocolate or anything containing sugar; salty savouries such as crisps, rich or heavy sauces.

10
Food and Mood

IF YOU ARE tired, upset, depressed or anxious without apparent cause, the problem could lie in your diet. Not only do some people appear to suffer from allergies to specific (sometimes even highly *nutritious*) foods which can set their mind and feelings whirling or make them depressed, an upset in the mineral balance in your body or low blood sugar can have similar consequences. For the foods you eat can exert powerful effects on your mind. On the positive side, scientists are beginning to investigate how foods, or the specific factors they contain, can be used to alter states of consciousness, to improve mood and to induce relaxation. Understanding how food may affect your own moods and mental states and learning how to make foods work *for* you in this way can be very useful to the ultrahealth player. Let's look at food allergies first.

Food on the Brain
In some medical circles the question of food allergies is still met with hostility – even scorn. For physicians and psychiatrists since Freud have believed that problems such as chronic anxiety, depression, hysteria, psychosomatic illnesses and other functional disorders arise almost entirely from psychogenic factors. Now, however, as the result of the work of biochemist and psychiatrist Dr. Abram Hoffer in Canada, American allergists Dr. Ted Randolph and Dr. Albert Rowe, British psychiatrist Dr. Richard Mackarness and others, it is beginning to look as though factors in our physical environment such as specific foods or chemicals in foods, air and water can be equally important in causing mental or emotional symptoms in some people by inducing sensitivity or allergic

reactions which involve the central nervous system. The study of this phenomenon is called clinical ecology.

For many years clinical ecologists have been testing patients with psychiatric problems or simple depression or anxiety to see if the cause of these things comes from food allergies. They either do this through a complicated procedure called cytotoxic testing – using blood from the patient and checking how it reacts to specific substances, or by putting the patient on a fast for five days and then introducing a drop of water containing the suspected food under the patient's tongue and charting his or her reactions. These include changes in pulse-rate and other physical symptoms and natural shifts of mood or emotional outbursts, indicating that this particular food is a troublemaker. Reactions vary from patient to patient – from something as simple as a feeling of mental confusion, grief or fatigue, to a dramatic psychopathic outburst in which the patient tries to slash his wrists or attack those testing him. Once the offending foods are known (they might be milk, grains, cheese, sugar – or almost anything) the patient is told to eliminate them from his diet. Provided he does so, his aberrant emotional or mental state does not recur. If the allergies are mild they can often be controlled by a 'rotation diet' in which food intake is carefully planned so that the person only eats a particular food once in any four-day period. Food allergies are far more common than most people realize. Two of the worst 'offenders' are wheat and milk products. Many people find that if they exclude these foods completely from their diet their energy levels increase and their disposition improves.

The Heavy Metal Problem
Heavy metals such as lead, mercury and cadmium, metals such as aluminium, or too high a concentration of copper (one of the trace minerals necessary for good health) in your body, can also interfere with the brain and central nervous system as well as the endocrine system and result in aberrant emotions. An excess of copper, for instance, can bring about hyperemotionalism, hallucinations and even psychic experiences. A high level of lead in the body has been linked to mental retardation in children and is often a significant factor in over-aggressive behaviour. It is also implicated as a cause of hyperactivity and learning problems in children. Excess

cadmium, from a lifestyle that includes taking several cups of coffee a day, often leads to a low blood-sugar problem so that you feel you need more coffee or something sweet just to keep going. Low blood-sugar is common amongst people living on a typical British or American diet. There are some simple tests to help determine mineral balance and the levels of heavy metals in your body, though these tests are not foolproof. They are done by burning a small sample of hair cut from the head and then analysing its mineral content. If any imbalances are found they can be corrected by giving chelated minerals or by drawing out excessive heavy metals from the tissues using natural substances such as pectin – a kind of fibre which occurs in apples – vitamin C, garlic, and kelp supplements.

The Mood Affectors

Quite apart from their ability to cause allergic or sensitive reactions, specific foods have tendencies to affect the human body and mind in very special ways, both mental and physical. Knowing just which does what can be useful when choosing your menus to improve your mood, alter your state of consciousness or help treat a specific problem such as overweight, poor nail and hair condition or cellulite in women. For instance, bananas contain tryptophan, a sleep-inducing amino acid that can have anti-depressant properties. Watermelons contain a natural diuretic which helps remove excess fluid from cellulite-prone bodies, as well as a complicated chemical, cucurocitrin, which reduces blood pressure. Yams contain a phytohormone chemically akin to oestrogen. Many experts in plant chemistry are convinced that women approaching menopause, or who have had a hysterectomy, can benefit from eating yams regularly. These are only three of the hundreds of foods whose chemical effects on mind and body are now recognized.

Beyond Nutrition

These chemical effects are quite separate from a food's nutritional properties. Indeed, many nutritionists show little understanding of the new research into plant chemistry: according to them, any plant which has a chemical effect must be classified as a drug, not as a food. But in reality the distinction between a plant as food and a plant-based drug is tenuous. The common spice, pepper, for instance, is both a stimulant and a mild euphoriant. So is nutmeg: in small quantities – a couple of cloves – it causes hallucination. Marijuana, peyote cactus (mescaline) and psilocybin mushrooms are also powerful consciousness- altering foods which we choose to call drugs, while white cabbage, which we tend to regard solely as a food, is used by some physicians in the United States and Russia to cure stomach ulcers and help alcoholics withdraw from their addiction. What is now clear is that certain foods, taken often, in large quantities or in combination with other foods, may alter one's personality, create feelings of elation or depression and even enhance creativity.

Some scientists such as George Schwartz MD, associated professor of medicine at the University of New Mexico, believe that eventually we will be able to modify behaviour and feelings through food alone. Schwartz spent over ten years researching food chemistry and comparing biochemical analyses of various foods with their reputed 'folk' properties. He first became interested in food effects when he observed that some foods eaten for breakfast would keep him bright and clear-headed all morning while others seemed to lull him into lethargy and make it difficult to work at all.

He began to investigate claims for a number of foods. He discovered that many old-fashioned ideas about how different foods affected us were true – chicken soup, for example, does contain substances helpful in treating a cold. (In fact many of the chemicals it contains are found in commercial 'cold remedies'.) In *Food Power* (McGraw-Hill, New York), Schwartz writes, 'Various cultures have recognized the power of foods and have developed diets for special purposes. Knowledge of the chemistry of foods sheds new light on the effectiveness of such diets and allows more respect and appreciation for the wisdom of the ancients. For example the spare diet or fasting of religious retreats tends to induce a more mystical state of mind. Fasting alters the body metabolism substantially, affecting the brain.' So, it appears, do a number of single foods.

Banishing Negative Emotions

Take pomegranates, for instance. The Buddha said, 'They will cleanse your soul of hatred and envy.' A chemical analysis of this complex fruit, which contains alkaloids of the pelleterine variety, reveals that some of these alkaloids are chemically akin to mescaline while others mimic the structure of the sedatives tryptophan and tryptamine. Tryptophan and tryptamine are involved in the production of the neurotransmitter serotonin in the brain. Serotonin levels have been correlated with tranquillity. The pomegranate is also a source of plant hormones akin to some female hormones which can cause personality alterations. Similarly, mangoes, which in Hindu tradition are considered 'fruits of heavenly joy', contain two compounds, anacardic acid and anacardiol, which are closely related chemically to some anti-depressant drugs. Carrots, which contain a hormone-like substance in their seeds, do appear to have aphrodisiac properties for women, just as the ancient Greeks claimed. Many vegetables, such as cabbage, broccoli and swede, have a mild thyroid-depressing action. Too many of them too often can make some people feel very 'down'.

Other vegetables, such as lettuce (which contains lactucin, a relaxation-inducing chemical) produce relaxation when eaten in quantity. When the leaves of the wild lettuce are dried, or when its juices are extracted, the resulting stuff can cause a drugged state. This is because wild lettuce and some other varieties contain hyoscyamine – a chemical similar to scopolamine, which was used on prisoners of war as 'truth serum' and on women during childbirth to distort their sense of time and to lessen awareness of pain. Horseradish contains sinigrin, a mild stimulant in low doses; parsley has apiol in it – a gentle sedative with aspirin-like effects; rosemary contains borneol, eucalyptol, and pinene and is a stimulant associated with improving memory. Fennel contains pinene and fenchone, both mild stimulants. Even the humble potato contains low levels of sleep-inducing scopolamine alkaloids.

Making Mind Foods Work for You

Great benefits can result if you take advantage of new knowledge in choosing the kind of meals you eat and in singling out specific foods which may be of particular help for certain problems. For instance, if in the middle of the day you find yourself feeling tired, you would do well to avoid foods which contain substances that encourage further relaxation at lunch. So instead of a large lettuce, radish and cabbage salad (all of which have sedative effects), you should choose a salad of sprouted seeds or grains, fresh spring onions, fennel and fish seasoned with rosemary (all contain stimulants).

If you have trouble keeping your weight down you might be wise to avoid eating large quantities of the vegetables which are known to have a natural thyroid-depressing action such as soya beans, cabbage and peas. Other plant foods offer exceptional chemical help for good looks. Here are four high-powered foods particularly good for losing weight, improving the condition of hair and skin and banishing cellulite in women: spirulina, beetroot, seaweed and celery.

Did You Know That?

- Beetroot can help protect from pollution-caused age-related damage to the body?

- Celery can help eliminate cellulite in a woman's body?

- Mangoes are a natural anti-depressant?

- Bananas and lettuce calm your nerves?

- Watermelon is a natural diuretic?

The Spirulina Factor

Spirulina, a blue-green algae, is higher in protein than almost any other food. This primitive single-celled plant, only visible through a microscope, contains high quantities of vitamin B (more than liver), betacarotene (from which the body makes vitamin A), iron and a number of other important trace elements. Its nutritional qualities are so exceptional that many food scientists believe that spirulina may hold a key to the world's food problems.

Spirulina is an excellent natural aid to fat-loss and appetite control. Unlike the 'bulking' products such as *carbodymethylcellulose* which rely on plumping up your stomach to make you feel less hungry, spirulina appears to have a direct chemical action on the brain's satiety centre, thus reducing appetite. The reason for this seems to be that spirulina is very high in one particular chemical – an amino acid called *phenylalanine* – which itself acts in the brain to suppress appetite. As an aid to weight-loss, spirulina tablets or capsules can be taken about twenty minutes before each meal. How much depends on individual body chemistry. (Because of its high phenylalanine content spirulina should not be taken by anyone with high blood pressure.) It is usually best to start with three 500 mg tablets before each meal and see how you get on. Some people find this is more than they need; others take as many as six or eight tablets at a time. There is no worry about taking too many since they are nothing more than the dried pressed plant; they are also an excellent source of protein.

Spirulina may also be of use to joggers. Many sportsmen take as much as eight grammes of the algae believing that it improves their endurance and helps prevent cramp. The reason for this is probably that spirulina contains a good quantity of ferredoxin, a chemical which helps the rapid elimination of carbon dioxide which can otherwise cause a breakdown of the saccharides in the muscles when one is strenuously exercising.

Beetroot Power

Beetroot can also be helpful for fat-loss. One of the major problems with anyone trying to lose weight, particularly if they have been overweight for some time, is mobilizing the fat which is stored in the body so that it can be burned as energy. Beetroot contains the alkaloid betaine, which has a significant action on the liver, helping to detoxify it, stimulating its normal function. It has long been used in folk remedies in France and Germany for treating liver problems. Unless your liver is working properly, fat cannot be efficiently broken down and transported through the body for use and elimination. A poorly functioning liver can result in bilious attacks, fatigue, illness and overweight. Raw beetroot juice, taken regularly, is believed to help spur fat mobilization as well as generally toning the whole body. A natural colourant which occurs in beetroot has also been shown to have anti-cancer and anti-ageing properties. You can make the juice in a juice extractor. If you find it too 'earthy' for your taste, try mixing it with apple or carrot juice. Beetroot juice specially prepared by a low-heat system to preserve the activities of its natural enzymes is also available from healthfood stores.

Seaweed and Good Looks

As well as being useful in the treatment of constipation, nervous troubles, arthritis, fatigue and skin irritations, sea plants are remarkable for the way in which they help produce luxuriant hair, strong nails and clear smooth skin. This is largely because they contain important minerals, proteins, trace elements and vitamins in an easily assimilable colloidal state. But it is probably the organic iodine (combined with other as yet unidentified chemicals in sea plants) which, because it can have such a strong effect on the metabolism, makes seaweeds so useful in mobilizing fat. Iodine is essential to the efficient function of the thyroid and parathyroid glands and, like some other plants, seaweeds appear to correct both overactivity and underactivity of the thyroid.

Since an underactive thyroid is very common amongst people over 35, and even more common in overweight people, sea plants such as kelp can often do a great deal to help them shed pounds and feel more energetic in the process. Kelp tablets are inexpensive and available from healthfood stores and chemists. Various types of sea plants for cooking can also be found in healthfood stores and oriental food shops.

Celery
Celery, traditionally a Hungarian gypsy remedy for skin troubles in both men and women, can also help women who want to eliminate cellulite. Its stem, leaves and seeds all contain active ingredients including apiol – a chemical often used by herbalists to treat or prevent colds and catarrh.

Long considered a folk remedy for arthritis and rheumatism, celery contains anti-inflammatory substances and has a strong diuretic power; both these characteristics can help banish cellulite. Celery's essential oil (which gives it its strong smell) also appears to have a highly beneficial effect on the nervous system. Like ginseng, it has tonic properties and yet at the same time calms the nerves. The best way to eat celery is raw, or by extracting the juice and mixing it with beetroot and carrot juices. Many of its health-giving properties are lost when the vegetable is heated.

These are only a few of the foods known to affect your body and your mood in particular ways. There are many more. One of the interesting things about ultrahealth eating is that when you rid your body of the effects of a high-fat, high-protein diet that includes refined processed foods you gradually become sensitive and aware enough to begin to chart your own 'mood affectors'. For everyone's body is unique – biochemically individual – and nobody reacts to a certain food exactly as someone else would. Eventually, by following the ultrahealth guidelines for diet, you should come to the point where you no longer need to think twice about whether or not a food is 'good' for you. A taste or a sniff of it will tell you all you need to know.

PART FOUR

MIND GAMES

11
The Mind-Body Dynamic

PSYCHOLOGICAL FACTORS PLAY as vital a part in ultrahealth as do the biochemical and neurophysiological influences that come from the foods you eat and the way you use your body. For the notion which most people have, that mind and body are separate entities – a philosophical model which goes back to Cartesian dualism, on which many of our common assumptions are based – no longer holds water. Research into biofeedback, the placebo effect, and the ability of the mind to induce measurable physiological changes in your body shows clearly that, far from being two separate entities, mind and body are better viewed as two ends of a continuum. They affect and influence each other in an almost infinite number of ways. So closely are they interrelated that to try and separate them in your thinking is to severely distort your awareness of either. When you feel happy and relaxed your body benefits. When you feel tense and worried it suffers in quite specific physiological ways. It works the other way round too. Many so-called psychological stages – from anxiety and depression to euphoria and transcendence – can be induced by specific foods and body chemicals. These 'moods' are also affected by different practices – from meditation to vigorous exercise. Much of human emotional behaviour can be traced to biochemical causes. The exact pathways of mind–body interaction are as yet only partially understood. Communication appears primarily to be mediated through the autonomic nervous system and the mid-brain; it seems to be highly dependent on the actions of pituitary hormones and of messenger chemicals or neurotransmitters. The latter, amongst other things, strongly influence behaviour, thoughts and feelings.

So potent is the effect of mind on body and body on mind that unless you have a positive attitude and a sense of enjoyment in life, and unless you are able successfully to manage stress, you are greatly undermining the potential you have for ultrahealth – regardless of how good the other dimensions for wellness in your life appear to be. To understand *why*, it is important you need to look at three things:

1. The concept of stress.
2. What is known about brain chemistry and behaviour.
3. Methods for taking control and directing your own life, rather than just going along with whatever happens. Let's look at stress first.

You Need Stress to Live

Without physical and mental challenges your body would become feeble and you would never feel the excitement and creative energy which are such an important part of ultrahealth. But too much stress can be a killer since stress, or rather the inability to cope with it, is the common denominator in all disease states. It is also a strong contributing cause in almost every illness to which we are susceptible. If you develop ultrahealth methods for neutralizing the negative effects of stress on your body, then you can begin to really benefit from its positive aspects.

Toss Out the Pills

Drug-based therapy is not the answer: the 650,000 tons of Valium consumed yearly in the world, like the huge quantities of sleeping pills and other tranquillizers, produce unpleasant and dangerous side-effects ranging from addiction to acute rage reactions, withdrawal, long-term worsening of anxiety symptoms, sub-clinical vitamin and mineral deficiencies, aggressiveness and even acute psychotic episodes. New evidence indicates that taking tran- quillizers may also encourage the growth of tumours, impair neuromuscular coordination and even make takers more prone to road accidents. But, quite apart from the detrimental effects of these drugs on your mind and body, the fact that they treat only the *symptoms* of stress overload and do absolutely nothing towards eliminating the *causes*, means they can never make a positive contribution to wellness. Perhaps most important of all to the ultrahealth player, relying on pills weakens your ability to cope with life and undermines your autonomy. But stress needn't be a negative force in your life. It can be a friend.

Quick Energy Trick

It is actually possible to breathe in energy. Try this for a couple of minutes:

Close your eyes and breathe slowly and deeply from your diaphragm, so your stomach (not your chest) swells with each inbreath. Imagine that you are breathing in vitality from the air to fill your whole body through your solar plexus. As you breathe in, feel that your whole body is becoming more and more relaxed. Imagine it as a centre of immense light radiating outward in all directions, as though you are taking in energy through the solar plexus itself, transforming it into light and radiating it out again everywhere.

What is Stress?

It is difficult to define: strain, fatigue, overwork, loss of blood, physical damage, grief and joy can all produce stress, but not one of them accurately describes what it is. The leader of a mountaineering team faced with a difficult ascent on which the lives of his or her group depend is under stress. So is the woman who burns her hand cooking and the child forced to walk home from school in the freezing rain. Although the conditions these people face are different and although each one's *specific* response varies (the mountaineer experiences sweating and tightness in the stomach, the woman shock and inflammation of her hand, the child shivering and pallor), they all respond in a stereotyped manner and undergo identical biochemical changes to help them cope with an increased demand on the organism. They all experience the same increased production of corticoid hormones and of adrenaline from the adrenal glands, and a number of other neurological, biochemical and physical changes which together make up the 'stress response'. Hans Selye has defined stress as 'the non-specific response of the body to any demand made upon it'. This is an important concept to grasp if you are to understand the ultrahealth approach to wellness and illness, but it is also a difficult concept. For it is funny to think that your body can respond to experiences as different as cutting your hand and hearing the news that you have just won the Irish

Sweepstake in exactly the same manner. But this has been demonstrated again and again in objective quantitative biochemical research. It is not the 'stressor' which causes problems such as illness, but the level of your ability to cope with it.

Selye's definition of stress is now accepted in many standard medical texts. The implication of these findings – that by being able to withstand stress (and by eliminating it when unnecessary) one can actually control the health of the body – is tremendously exciting. For it means that we are not doomed to inevitable illness later in life; nor to the premature ageing we now see around us, which adversely affects the cardiovascular system, the endocrine glands and the look of your skin. To quote the journal of the American Medical Association: 'Nature did not intend us to grow old and ill; we were designed to die young in old age but free of disease.'

The Art of Sighing

When you begin to unwind and let go the muscles' tension, the release is often accompanied by a very slow deep breath – in fact, a sort of sigh. You can use sighing throughout the day to calm your nerves and prevent tensions building up. Think of a stress-producing situation which occurs fairly frequently at work, e.g. the telephone ringing, and each time it happens, take a deep breath and let it out again, then answer the phone.

Be sure to let your shoulders drop as you inhale and breathe deeply down into your belly and lower back. Let the lower ribs expand away from your spine as much behind as in front. When you exhale, don't collapse, but think of your head and spine lengthening upwards.

The Stress Reaction

The stereotyped reactions characteristic of stress are known as the 'general adaptation syndrome' or GAS. The purpose of GAS is to maintain the structure and function of your body in a steady state – known as homeostasis – and by doing so to preserve your life. Every 'stressor' with which you come into contact threatens to some degree to destroy homeostasis. The moment this happens GAS goes into action. GAS has three recognizable stages: an initial *alarm* or alerting reaction, a stage of active *resistance*, and a stage of *exhaustion*. During the alarm reaction, when GAS is first set in motion, your overall resistance is lowered, the sympathetic nervous system fires, brainwaves change, muscles tense, peripheral circulation increases and the adrenals secrete hormones more rapidly. During the resistance stage, all your body's systems are stimulated into increased activity in order to meet the challenge presented and to protect it from harm – in effect your resistance is raised. This stage can last for a short or long while, depending on your individual make-up and on the intensity of your reaction to the stressor. But it cannot go on forever. Sooner or later the third stage is reached – exhaustion. Your body's weakest systems break down, chronic fatigue and illness follow. If this exhaustion stage of GAS continues the body eventually dies.

Each Person is Unique

Every individual differs in his or her reaction to stressors (a stressor to one person may not be one to another, although certain stressors, such as burning, affect everyone), and in how much stress you can take before reaching the exhaustion stage. This depends on conditioning and on the amount of adaptive energy you are born with. Researchers still do not precisely understand adaptive energy. It is not the same as caloric energy, which can be replaced by food. One person will have a great deal – he or she may be on the move constantly and may be able to withstand a great deal of stress, while another, when faced with the same stress, quickly reaches the GAS exhaustion stage. As Selye used to say: 'If you are a racehorse you have to be a racehorse but if you are a turtle and you try to be a racehorse you asking for trouble.' The point is that once your adaptive energy is used up as a result of the wear and tear of stress, nothing can be done to restore it. This makes it imperative to examine carefully how it is being used in your own life and to question if it is being used up unnecessarily. It also means that you can benefit from becoming aware of your own stress patterns and optimum stress levels, remembering that it is as bad for a racehorse to be made to function as a turtle as it is for a turtle to be pushed into behaving like a racehorse.

Lack of stress can also be a stressor. Not only is it impossible for you to avoid all stress, but it would be a highly undesirable state to live in, even if you could. For the drive which makes life refreshing and which makes art, discoveries and inventions possible owes a lot to the hormonal and nervous changes which are part of the stress GAS reaction. One of the most important mind/body keys to long-lasting health and good looks is to learn to use stress to your advantage.

Making Stress Work for You

The first step is to examine how you may be wasting your adaptive energy by putting yourself under unnecessary stress. By identifying the unnecessary stressors and eliminating them you free a lot of energy for more positive use and for meeting important challenges.

Many of the ingredients in a high-energy way of living such as the ultrahealth diet, and regular aerobic exercise do this for you automatically. For instance, physical inactivity is a serious stressor. It decreases your body's ability to function at optimal levels, encourages muscle shrinkage and the decrease in hormonal secretions that accompany it, depletes you of valuable minerals, encourages the storage of wastes in muscles and skin and makes you feel chronically fatigued. An active lifestyle not only eliminates the serious stressor of inactivity from which most people suffer, it also improves your ability to cope with stress in other ways too. Taking the time to participate in some physical activity reflects a particular psychological attitude to yourself and your body – an attitude which will lead you to react in new, more positive ways in your work and your relationships with other people. It can even alter your personal values. People who take up regular exercise often experience 'conceptual shifts' so that things which appeared stressful before no longer upset them. That woman on the bus every morning who has for weeks been raising your blood pressure by humming the same tune under her breath suddenly no longer bothers you. She becomes an object of pity or amusement to you, rather than one of your stressors.

Like cigarettes and drugs, various foods and drinks are heavy stressors. They offer nothing in the way of positive health and vitality, but instead are a constant drain on your body's adaptive energy. It is well established that caffeine, alcohol, tobacco, excess fat and sugar are stressors. Excess protein too has recently come under attack. They are things your body not only doesn't need, but which actively work against its normal healthy functioning. That's why an ultrahealth lifestyle eliminates them.

Jet Setting without Jet Lag

The Problem: *Circadian dysrhythmia* or *desynchronosis* – one of the worst stresses your body can be subjected to.
The Cause: Travel across four time zones or more at a speed in excess of 400 mph.
The Symptoms: Exhaustion, depression and mood swings, confusion, sleeplessness at night, headaches, loss of appetite at meal times, cravings between meals, constipation, peptic ulcers, reduction in REM sleep, disruption of body temperature.
Additional side-effects of jet travel: General dehydration, dry skin.

Prescription

- Get plenty of exercise before flight.
- Eat only light foods such as salads and fruit the day before a flight and then fast on juice or just eat fruit during the flight itself. On many long flights you can actually order a 'fruitarian' meal. Let the airlines know 24 hours in advance that you have special dietary requirements.

  Research shows that people who eat very little during a flight suffer considerably less from jet lag symptoms because they do not have to adjust their eating patterns to fit a new schedule. They simply set up a new digestive cycle by eating a light meal at a local meal-time once they arrive at their destination and then avoid heavy foods for the next couple of days until their bodies have had time to adjust.

- Take a night flight if possible – avoid the evening meal and sleep through (see natural tranquillizers pages 117–18 and relaxation techniques page 159).

- Drink water or fruit/vegetable juices to restore body fluids which are lost very quickly in the dry cabin air.

- Avoid alcohol – its effects are twice as potent in a plane. It also interferes with your body's ability to use oxygen.

- Take stress vitamin and mineral supplements (see pages 135–6) during the flight and for at least the first few days of your stay.

- Take 15 mg of melatonin at 8pm for four days before the flight and five days afterwards to help regulate circadian rhythms.

- Sit in the 'no smoking' section. Cigarette smoke is particularly irritating to the mucous membranes in the throat, sinuses and eyes in the dry cabin air.

- If possible get up and stretch your legs and back by walking up and down the aisle a couple of times to get your circulation going and help eliminate cellular wastes.

- Replenish the moisture lost from your face by using a good moisturizing cream.

Your Feelings Matter

Emotional stressors in your life also take their toll. But for most people, many emotional hurdles can be overcome. Take a look at what continues to trigger off the stress response in your life and ask yourself whether it is something which prevents you from turning a lot of your energy to more constructive use. Some stressors provide challenges from which you can grow. Others are simply habitual. They lead nowhere and bring little in terms of increasing your awareness or your ability to make better use of your energy. If there are any of these in your life perhaps you can eliminate them. For instance, take a look at the work you do and ask yourself if you find it really satisfying. Are the financial responsibilities you have taken on really necessary? Can you reduce them in any way? If so, have the courage to drop them and to accept the changes this will bring about; that too can make you stronger. We all have a tendency to hang on to the status quo at all costs – and often the cost is in terms of lost adaptive energy – occasionally even life. Regardless of whether you learn the world's finest techniques for meditation to counteract stress, if you are in a job you hate year after year or are faced with a relationship that no longer has meaning for you, they will do little good. To make stress work you must not only face up to its demands, but also take responsibility for removing it wherever it is no longer useful and relevant to you.

Create a Balance

Learning a technique for conscious relaxation and practising it regularly is one of the most potent actions you can take for eliminating excess stress because it restores your body's equilibrium and homeostasis. When stress occurs, a group of nerve fibres radiating from the spinal cord and linked with *catecholamines* or the adrenaline class of hormones respond. They are concerned with energy expenditure – particularly the energy involved with the stress reaction. They spur your heart to beat faster, make you breathe harder, encourage sweating and raise your blood pressure. They also inhibit the secretion of gastric juices and digestion and send blood to your muscles. These nerve fibres are known as the *sympathetic* branch of the autonomic nervous system.

The other branch – the *parasympathetic* – is made up mostly of nerve fibres from the tenth cranial or vagus nerve. Its activity is linked with the acetylcholine class of hormones. This branch is concerned with rest rather than action. In fact, the parasympathetic action works more or less in direct opposition to that of the sympathetic: it slows your heart-rate, reduces the flow of air to your lungs, stimulates your digestive system and urges your muscles to relax. Where the sympathetic reaction puts wear and tear on your body, the parasympathetic restores it. A good balance between the two is the key to enormous energy. When you are able to move freely at will from one to the other – from the active stressed state to the passive relaxed one – then your body maintains its equilibrium with relative ease and homeostasis is never severely threatened, regardless of what stressors you confront.

You Are in Control

The autonomic nervous system was once thought to be outside your control, and the bodily functions – such as heartbeat, temperature, and so forth, which it governs – entirely automatic. But studies have shown that human beings can be relatively easily taught to exercise a high level of control over the autonomic nervous system. You can learn to release excessive nervous and physical tension and to move from the active stressed state to the passive relaxed one at will. Learning and using this skill significantly reduces the psychological and physical effects of stress on your body and preserves your adaptive energy. Moreover, it creates a balance which enables you to go out into the world to do, to make, to create, to fight and to express, as well as to retire into yourself to regenerate, to rest, to recuperate and to enjoy and to find the space for discovering new ideas and planting the seeds of future actions.

Learning to move from stress to relaxation and back again is not difficult. You can achieve it by taking up forms of meditation or deep relaxation. When practised regularly they help make you no longer prey to the kind of internal stress response that can literally kill you. Here are a few useful tools:

Transcendental Commuting
One of the most stressful parts of any working person's day is 'rush hour'. No matter how well you feel, the hustle and bustle amongst crowds of tired or irritable people can leave you drained. Here are a few simple tricks to counter 'rush-houritis':

Breathing on the Bus
A quick energy pick-up you can do on a crowded bus or train, provided you have a seat, is to close your eyes and release the tensions in your body. Then listen to the sounds around you and, if they seem irritating, try to focus or 'pan-in' on one particular noise at a time, excluding the others. Then gradually let the sounds become 'background' and focus on your breathing. Watch yourself take an 'in breath' and then an 'out breath'. At the end of each out breath repeat a word silently in your mind such as 'one' or 'peace' or 'calm'. Repeat the breathing for five minutes or so and then gently open your eyes. Your mind will be clear and you will feel rested.

Singing in the Car
If you travel to work by car try turning on the radio or playing a favourite cassette and singing along. Singing (whether it's melodic or croak-like) is amazingly therapeutic and does wonders to lift your spirits and boost your energy level.

Sighing on the Tube
If you have to put up with the misery of standing in a tightly packed tube or bus, one of the best things you can do is to breathe deeply and avoid tensing your body. Try imagining that you have roots growing down through the soles of your feet (especially the heels). Then imagine the top of your head lifting up towards the sky. These two simple visualizations will realign your spine and make it

possible for you to breathe deeply from your lower abdomen without lifting or tensing your shoulders.

Create a Personal Lifestyle for Stress Management

Everybody needs to develop his own personal ways of throwing off stress. A walk in the woods for clearing consciousness is something quite specifically ordered by Tibetan doctors to patients who suffer from rapid swings of mood and worry. Or you could try sailing, running, dancing, gardening, listening to music or some other form of hobby. Explore them all. Find out what works best for you and make it an important part of your day-to-day life. By eliminating unnecessary stressors from your life, practising relaxation and exercise, and becoming more and more aware of which challenges are important to you and which you are better off without, you will rapidly progress towards ultrahealth and you will also develop a lifestyle which will keep you free from illness. You will soon be tapping the kind of vitality and enthusiasm a child has which most adults have long forgotten. A special bonus too – you will quite automatically preserve your youthful contours and smooth clear skin, decade after decade.

Anti-Stress Vitamins and Minerals

Do you suffer from vitamin and mineral deficiencies? Many people do. The problem is discovering which ones. Unless you go through the lengthy and often expensive process of having a mineral hair and blood analysis done, the best way to discover the answer is by the process of probability.

- Do you eat any of the following vitamin and mineral depletors: coffee, sugar, alcohol, refined foods?

- Do you take: antibiotics, aspirin, cortisone, sulphur drugs, birth control pills, laxatives, excessive amounts of salt?

- Do you smoke?

- Are you exposed to other high stress factors?

If the answer is yes to even a few of these questions, then it is likely that you will be deficient in one or more of the water-soluble vitamins and minerals – those easily depleted by stress – including:

vitamin C, B complex vitamins, calcium, potassium, magnesium and zinc. To boost your system for coping with everyday stress or to help deal with extraordinary situations – overwork, jet lag, worry etc., you might consider taking a special anti-stress supplement which contains the following nutrients:

Vitamin C	1,000mg
B1	50mg
B2	50mg
B3	25mg
B6	50mg
Pantothenic acid	50mg
Folic acid	400mcg
B12	20mcg
B15	30mg
Choline	250mg
Inositol	250mg
PABA	100mg
Biotin	50mcg
Calcium	1,000mg
Magnesium	500mg
Zinc	50mg
Potassium	25–50mg

(Nutritional experts usually recommend that their patients take such supplements three times a day with meals.)

Bubble Bath
A warm bath enriched with a few drops of your favourite bath gel is one of the greatest luxuries after a hard day's work. Here is a simple technique you can use in the bath to help let go of any tensions and float your worries away . . .

- Lie down in a warm bath (not scorching hot) with a rubber bath pillow or improvised towel-pillow under your head.

- Close your eyes and take a nice big SIGH.

- Let go of any tension in your forehead and the rest of your body.

- Allow your breathing to become steady and calm.

- Now imagine any thoughts, worries, problems, as bubbles which float up and out of your consciousness and fade into the distance. Each bubble can have a label, e.g. 'Bills'. By watching it you acknowledge it and then let it drift out of your mind.

- Gradually the bubbles come more slowly until you are left with a still, clear mind.

- You will be free from the niggling worries that plague you and have a chance to rest deeply.

- When you are ready, gradually open your eyes.

- Get out of the bath slowly and dry yourself; then massage some oil into your skin.

- Emerge rested and refreshed to face the evening ahead or whatever things need your attention. They are infinitely easier to deal with without anxiety and tension.

12
The Chemistry of Consciousness

IN CHARLES DICKENS' *A Christmas Carol*, Jacob Marley, Scrooge's dead partner, appears to him as a ghost:

> 'You don't believe in me,' observed the Ghost. 'I don't,' said Scrooge. 'What evidence would you have of my reality beyond that of your senses?' 'I don't know,' said Scrooge. 'Why do you doubt your senses?' 'Because', said Scrooge, 'a little thing affects them. A slight disorder of the stomach makes them cheat. You may be an undigested bit of beef, a blot of mustard, a crumb of cheese, a fragment of an underdone potato. There's more of gravy than of grave about you, whatever you are!'

Scrooge in his wisdom (even back in 1843!) well knew that biochemical changes brought about by something you eat can affect your brain and alter consciousness enough to produce imaginary fears and even hallucinations. But, thanks to several generations of 'psychologically-oriented' doctors influenced by Freudian theories, only recently have top scientists begun to chart the exact mechanisms of how, *via* your brain, biochemistry alters perceptions. We have long regarded the brain as the centre for thought, emotion, mood perception, drive and memory, yet we often overlook the fact that it also produces an abundance of important hormones and other chemicals which are largely responsible for altering the pattern of its functions and for changing the way you think, feel and perceive your world. Joy, paranoia – even despair – can all be related to the delicate balance (or imbalance) of these potent chemical substances. If, as many researchers now believe, we can learn to influence this balance without causing adverse side-effects (such as those which result from the use of tranquillizers, anti-depressant drugs or sleeping pills), then we will be able to exercise greater control over destructive moods and feelings and increase our enjoyment of life considerably. Such thinking has something to offer the ultrahealth player.

Chemical Brain Power

Your brain weighs about three pounds. It is the most complex structure known to science in the entire universe. Next to it even the most advanced computer resembles a primitive abacus. Within the three pounds of grey material are woven tens of billions of nerve cells. Called neurons, they are embedded in a matrix of many more billions of supporting cells. Each of these nerve cells is bathed in a fluid which brings nourishment and oxygen to it and which eliminates wastes. And each is independently capable of making connections with hundreds, maybe even thousands of others in an organic system of extraordinary complexity.

Many brain researchers believe these inter-cell connections in the brain nerve network hold the essence of all brain functions from intellectual thought and emotions to blood-pressure control. Aberrations in them also appear to be responsible for much mental illness and changes in them to play a central part in ageing and its associated disorders such as loss of memory, a slowing down of the thinking processes, a tendency to depression and poor muscle control. Exciting new research has led many scientists to believe that by manipulating chemicals in the brain such degenerative age-changes might be postponed indefinitely. Some of them may even be reversible. Researchers are also uncovering biochemical ways of increasing intelligence, improving memory, calming hyperactivity in children and banishing depression by simple methods involving the use of nutritional supplements – vitamins, minerals and free amino acids – or even by using equipment for ionizing the air. To understand how chemical factors, nutritional supplements and various practices such as meditation and vigorous physical workouts can alter your moods, feelings and intellectual activity, you need first to know a little about how inter-cell connections are made.

The All-Powerful Neurotransmitters

Neurons communicate with each other by a combination of electrical and chemical signals in a complex series of events. Unlike most body cells, nerve cells are not round and compact. Instead they have long tendrils or shoots which radiate in all directions. These tendrils make contact with other cells and connect with them through the minute gaps which separate them, called synapses. The event begins with a change in the electrical potential of a cell membrane. This causes a tiny pulse of electric current to race down a nerve fibre towards the synapse, where it triggers the cell to release a special chemical messenger – called a neurotransmitter (NT) – into the synaptic cleft between the nerve tendril and the neighbouring cell on which it is resting. The membrane of the receiving cell has receptors which are able to recognize the substance being released and to bind themselves to it.

This act of receiving and binding in turn sets off a response in the receiving cell. Sometimes it is excitatory – triggering another electrical discharge. At other times it is inhibitory, in which case it suppresses the spontaneous electrical firing of the cell. The response depends on what kind of NT is released, and probably also on the cell receiving it. This complex process in fact happens almost simultaneously in your brain billions of times every day. So important is it that, in effect, your brain only works because these NTs make it possible for your nerve cells to 'talk to one another'.

NTs have become the subject of some of the most fascinating biological research in the world. In 1950 only five NTs were known. Now there are about 40. There may still be a hundred or more as yet undiscovered. Every mind-altering drug from sleeping pills to anti-depressants, from tranquillizers to LSD, almost certainly works by acting on one or more NTs or on the receptors to which they are directed. How well your brain functions, how you behave, your mood – even the way you feel about yourself and your life – are all intricately bound up with the working of your neurotransmitters.

The Diet Connection

These NTs are made by the brain out of nutrients from the foods you eat. There is strong evidence, thanks to the pioneering work of scientists in the field such as Richard Wurtman at MIT (the world expert in the link between brain biochemistry and behaviour), that at least five of the most important known NTs are directly diet-dependent: serotonin, acetylcholine, and the three catecholamines (adrenaline, noradrenaline and dopamine). In other words, levels of these neurotransmitters in the brain appear to be largely dependent on how much of the specific nutrients (amino acids) necessary for their manufacture (called precursors) are supplied in your diet. They vary dramatically depending on what kind of foods your body is digesting at any particular moment. For instance eating a high-carbohydrate, low-protein meal favours the uptake of tryptophan by your brain. Tryptophan is a precursor to one of the inhibitory neurotransmitters called serotonin, which is important for relaxation and for inducing sleep. Many people, particularly those over forty, have a deficiency of serotonin and suffer from a kind of physical restlessness which makes falling asleep difficult. A small carbohydrate snack at bedtime – perhaps a piece of wholegrain bread spread with a little cheese (which contains good quantities of tryptophan) can send them off to blissful slumber. A high-protein meal on the other hand has the opposite effect on serotonin production in the brain. It will lower serotonin levels and also tends to increase tyrosine, a precursor nutrient which stimulates the synthesis of the catecholamine NTs.

The Aggression Catecholamines

The catecholamines, if you remember from the last chapter, are the NTs associated with the energetic 'stressed' state. They are much more inclined to make you mentally active. Your body manufactures many of the catecholamine NTs, among them dopamine and noradrenaline, from a single amino acid, tyrosine. These two, together with adrenaline, affect your feelings of power, control and domination. Although they are different in their molecular structure and carry out different functions, they are very closely related chemically – so closely related, in fact, that each can actually be turned into the other in the brain when necessary. These catecholamines are important in regulating a wide variety of functions in your body, such as the workings of the limbic system or reptilian brain (that very old part of your brain which mediates primitive emotions and drives such as sex). They also determine how aggressive you are, help focus your concentration and can bring confidence. In a healthy person they are in a delicate balance with each other. When they become imbalanced this can lead to disturbed behaviour patterns. For instance, in very aggressive people levels of noradrenaline tend to be very low while those of dopamine are high. In schizophrenics the balance between dopamine and noradrenaline is even more severely disturbed. On the positive side, high levels of adrenaline improve the memory and both noradrenaline and adrenaline can make you more alert. Even whether or not you dream can depend on how much noradrenaline you have in your brain, for it also triggers the dream-producing neurons.

Nutritional Help for the Overactive Mind

American expert in vitamin and mineral therapy the late Dr. Carl Pfeiffer often used doses of vitamins to treat acute symptoms. He claimed that vitamin B3 and vitamin C taken together even in small quantities can provide almost instant relief to an overactive mind by focusing mental concentration. He used a combination of zinc, vitamin B6, and manganese to relieve the moody and fatiguing symptoms of low blood-sugar. He favoured such methods because unlike aspirin which erode the lining of your stomach, or tranquillizers which can create serious side-effects, these nutrients have neither immediate nor long-term adverse effects.

Training Heightens Noradrenaline

Dr. Robert S. Brown at the University of Virginia School of Medicine compared the psychological effects of physical training on normal and depressed patients. His studies showed that depressed patients experienced an alleviation of anxiety and got rid of their 'blues' after eight to ten weeks of jogging three times a week. The exercise was found to have brought about an elevation of the levels of noradrenaline in the brain and feelings of wellbeing which accompany it.

Lecithin Heightens Intelligence

Another example of the food–brain connection is the effect that a meal rich in lecithin (one containing liver or eggs for instance) can have. Lecithin raises blood and brain choline levels and increases acetylcholine synthesis in active neurons. It can make you feel particularly alert. Of course, all of these effects have been tested on people who eat the foods on an empty stomach. A meal which contains liver, but also such foods as potatoes, bread and sugar is unlikely to have the same effect. The important point is that science is beginning to demonstrate strong correlations between foods, herbal remedies, and specific nutrients and quantifiable mental or emotional states. Researchers have found that they can induce sleep, mood changes, pain sensitivity, selective appetite performance, physical activity and even social interactions between people by external means. They have tested valerian, for instance – one of the traditional herbal remedies for tension – and found that it does indeed improve the quality of sleep by its action on the brain. They have discovered that women tend to get sleepier after a carbohydrate meal than after a protein meal, while their male counterparts tend to experience only a pleasant calmness following a carbohydrate meal. And that depression in many people can be dramatically improved by feeding them nutrients such as the amino acids L-tyrosine and phenylalanine, which increase the levels of the NTs noradrenaline and dopamine.

Meals and Moods

Since tryptophan is used by the brain (together with vitamin B6, niacin and magnesium) to make serotonin, it can be helpful in alleviating anxiety states, depression and insomnia. It also appears useful in assisting alcoholics to remain dry. Cheese, bananas and turkey – all rich in tryptophan – must be taken together with a carbohydrate food – say wholegrain bread – in order to be turned into serotonin for brain use.

A high-protein meal *stimulates* you by increasing tyrosine levels and triggering catecholamine production.

Eating foods high in lecithin such as liver or eggs increases acetylcholine in your brain and can make you more *alert*.

The Migraine Connection

Migraine headaches can be triggered by an excess of certain NT precursor nutrients such as tyramine. Mature cheeses, wines, beers, yogurt, meat and yeast extracts, coffee, chocolate and tinned fish all contain tyramine which is absorbed through the blood-brain barrier into the brain. Many people who are susceptible to migraines find they have fewer headaches if they steer clear of these foods.

Acetylcholine, Sex, and Memory

The NT acetylcholine is used by the brain particularly for control of sensory input signals and muscular output. It is made from the precursor nutrient, choline. One of the B group of vitamins, choline not only occurs in liver and eggs, it is particularly rich in the dietary supplement lecithin, which is often taken to help control the level of fats in the blood. Another B vitamin, pantothenic acid, is needed for choline to be converted into acetylcholine in the body. This NT also plays an important part in your brain's memory functions and in the control of appetite and sex drives, as well as in mediating your responses to the environment. Low acetylcholine levels are, at least in part, responsible for the flagging sex interest in some people as they get older and for their lack of ability to concentrate. And very low levels of this NT are found in old people who cannot coordinate their movements properly.

Richard Wurtman and his colleagues at MIT did some interesting research on university students using choline supplements. They found it was possible to increase intelligence and memory by giving them three grammes of the vitamin a day. Other researchers have discovered that hyperactivity in children can be calmed and their concentration improved by increasing their choline intake.

Air Ions Affect Your Mind

Air ions – positively and negatively charged gas molecules in the air – affect serotonin levels in the brain. Negative ions – which are abundant in fresh air, particularly by the sea and in the mountains – help make you serene and calm but, at the same time, clear headed. They do this partly by balancing serotonin levels.

In polluted cities and offices, where positive ions are dominant, you are far more likely to suffer from low levels of serotonin and to become depressed and irritable.

An ionizer on your desk, by the side of your bed at night, or in your car if you do a lot of driving, can greatly alleviate such symptoms. Ionizers are also useful for people with respiratory difficulties and for some kinds of migraine.

Serotonin for Sound Sleep

Unlike acetylcholine, serotonin is inhibitory instead of stimulating in its actions. Instead of speeding up the activity of neurons, its function is to slow them down. That is why it is important in relaxing your body enough to send you to sleep. When the vitamins involved in serotonin production in the brain are given in good quantities, they encourage its production. (This is one of the reasons why doctors now prescribe vitamin B6 supplements to ease pre-menstrual tension.) Just before a period, as a result of hormonal changes in a woman's body, levels of serotonin drop and vitamin B6 helps rebalance them. Your body also uses this NT to fine tune your appetite. Tryptophan (as mentioned earlier), an amino acid which occurs in good quantity in milk, cheese and bananas, is its precursor. When well supplied to the brain it will be turned into serotonin. In fact there are several sleeping tablets on the market such as Optimax, Pacitron, and Trofan which are simply tryptophan. You can also buy it in health-food stores. But why then can't people just drink more milk in order to sleep better?

The Blood-Brain Barrier

Things are not quite so simple. The precursor nutrients, many of which are free amino acids (that is not bound together to make up long-chain proteins), have a superb ability to get through the blood-brain barrier – that membrane which helps protect your brain from damage. But just because you eat a food rich in a particular amino acid precursor, it doesn't mean that it will reach your brain for use in NT manufacture. Amino acids tend to compete with one another for brain entry. Many are also used up rapidly by the body for tissue repair before they even get the chance to become part of your brain's materials. That is why, in the clinical work which is being done to retard brain ageing and to treat emotional and mental troubles with precursor nutrients, they are usually given on their own, together with whatever vitamins or minerals are needed for their conversion. They are also usually given on an empty stomach, since more is made directly available for brain use this way. Tryptophan is special, however, in that it is more easily turned into serotonin when it is eaten together with carbohydrate foods – hence the biscuits and milk before bedtime and the suggestion by the doctor that you take tryptophan tablets together with a piece of bread.

NTs and Combating the Ageing Process

As you age, there is a decline in these chemical messengers in your brain. You make less of them, and you also become less responsive to their effects. What the new research shows, however, is that such a decline is not an inevitable part of growing older. New studies into the biochemistry of the brain and its effect on behaviour present strong evidence that various nutritional substances, such as certain free amino acids and some vitamins, may even help slow your brain's ageing process by providing adequate raw materials for making NTs. Some age-researchers claim that by using these precious nutrients, they are able to restore an aged brain. Another case for treatment is when someone is forgetful or depressed; certain NTs may restore him/her to more youthful functioning. A few of these precursors are also showing themselves to be helpful in improving the intelligence of normal young people. Others are now being used to treat various mental problems – from serious endogenous depression and schizophrenia to addiction anxiety states and even simple forms of fatigue or the 'blues'.

Appetite Suppressant

Another essential amino acid, phenylalanine, is also turned into NTs in the brain. It has a stimulating effect on the mental processes. It is used as a nutritional supplement to suppress the appetite, to increase mental alertness, and generally to improve your feeling of energetic wellbeing.

Phenylalanine is found in good quantity in almonds, pumpkin, sesame seeds, cottage cheese and lima beans and is most rich of all in spirulina. Here again this free amino acid should never be taken on its own by anyone with high blood pressure.

The Immune System and NTs

The catecholamines are particularly relevant to the ageing process in two ways. First, when there is a decline in them, you get the kind of loss of motivation and enthusiasm which many people begin to experience in middle age and which tends to worsen as the years pass. Second, this group of NTs also regulates the level of growth hormones in the body, which in turn are partly responsible for the healthy functioning of the immune system.

When growth hormones decline, the immune system's ability to resist infections and to protect the integrity of its cells also appears to fall off. The body becomes increasingly susceptible to ageing, cancer, and arteriosclerosis plaques. Some age researchers believe that certain free amino acids can be used to stimulate the production of these catecholamines, sometimes with remarkable results. For instance phenylalanine (usually taken with vitamin B6 and vitamin C, which are necessary for converting it into NTs) has shown itself to be useful in increasing inadequate levels of these catecholamines in the brain – another common contributor to depression. Two specific forms of other amino acids, L-ornithine and L-arganine, are also used to stimulate the production of growth hormones in the body and, claim some age researchers, by strengthening the immune system can protect the brain and body from age-related changes.

A New Class of Supernutrients

The use of free amino acids is an exciting development in clinical nutrition. These 'building-block' molecules from which proteins are made have extraordinary qualities when used on their own as nutritional supplements and therapeutic agents. They are currently being used to treat a wide variety of disease conditions, such as food allergies and addictions to alcohol and drugs, acute kidney failure and even jet lag and the stress of flying in outer space.

Each amino acid appears to have its own specific applications. For instance, lysine, one of the essential amino acids which your body cannot synthesize, is being used by nutritionally-oriented physicians in Britain and the United States as a remarkably effective treatment against the herpes virus. (Herpes is virtually impossible to treat with conventional methods.)

Other amino acids are being used to treat people with toxic levels of heavy metals in their system. The sulphur-bearing amino acids such as methionine, cystine and cysteine appear to act as natural chelating agents for mercury, lead, aluminium, cadmium and other toxic materials in the body, leaching them from the tissues in which they are stored and eliminating them via the bloodstream. Free amino acids have also been widely used in aerospace programmes in Russia and America where, in a balanced formula, they form the basis of astronauts' foods on space flights.

L-Glutamine – Brain Nutrient

Glutamic acid is another amino acid which appears essential to the proper functioning of the brain. Scientists now using it as a nutritional supplement in the form of L-glutamine have found it to have remarkable properties. It appears able to improve intelligence, speed up the healing of ulcers, lift fatigue, help control alcoholism and even schizophrenia. Because the biochemistry of NT production is so complex, and because glutamic acid does not directly cross the blood-brain barrier, eating large quantities of food containing it will not increase the amount present in your brain. But glutamic acid is readily made from L-glutamine, which passes into the brain and can be taken as a nutritional supplement. Abram Hoffer, Canadian expert on the treatment of mental conditions with therapeutic doses of nutritional supplements, has had success using glutamine in combination with other nutrients to treat senility and mental retardation, while another orthomolecular physician, H. L. Newbold, recommends it for general use in helping to fight fatigue, depression and impotence. Students taking exams claim that L-glutamine helps them think more clearly and improves their memories.

Approach with Caution

All of these nutrients which are precursors to the NTs are available in sophisticated healthfood stores and chemists. Although these nutrients are simply substances found in the foods we eat, to use them requires considerable knowledge. You really need the help of a nutritionally-oriented physician to make safe and effective use of them on their own as supplements. You also need to take into account what other nutrients – vitamins and minerals – work with them in NT conversions and to be aware of what precautions need to be taken when using them. The whole process of manipulating NTs for the purpose of improving brain functions, combating ageing and altering mood is something that as yet is little understood by the average doctor. But the promise they hold of being able to alter emotion and retard brain degeneration safely and simply appears extraordinary. In another fifteen years they are likely to become a part of the average GP's repertoire. Now they are one of the most sophisticated tools of the avant-garde scientist concerned with a biochemical approach to the mind-body continuum – and something anyone wanting to pursue an ultra-health lifestyle should know about.

13
Mind Power

POSSIBLY THE SINGLE most important dimension to ultrahealth is that of mind. A positive mental state full of images of high-level wellness, success and satisfaction can not only promote healing, it can also spur you towards the peaks of energy and good looks and keep you there. This notion, once considered the invention of weird 'success salesmen', is now becoming a respectable part of accepted medical opinion thanks to the large number of studies carried out in recent years showing how negative emotions exacerbate illnesses and how positive attitudes help restore health.

Western medicine has long acknowledged that negative states of mind, such as anxiety or depression, are important factors in the genesis of illnesses like tuberculosis, diabetes, asthma, ulcerative colitis, peptic ulcers and cardiovascular disorders. But, until recently, it has tended to pay little attention to the psychological components of these diseases. Now the relationship between the state of your mind and the ability of your body to protect you against illness has been well established. A study carried out in one of the leading medical schools in the United States, on more than 900 graduates spanning some 16 years, demonstrated that people who suffer feelings of isolation and have little sense of closeness to their parents as children have a significantly higher incidence of cancer than the rest. Those who tend to experience anxiety, nervous tension, and anger under stress have a higher incidence of coronary disease.

Placebos and the Mind-Body Interactions for Wellness
Other studies demonstrate that your state of mind, the way you

think about yourself, and how you view your future strongly influence recovery from illness. The use of placebos, whether fake drugs or mock operations, which have no power in themselves to heal but which the patient believes will do him or her good, has shown itself to be a potent method of healing in double blind tests. Scientists are even beginning to penetrate the mystery of how placebos work and are beginning to discover specific ways in which thoughts and emotions influence the biochemistry of ageing and your health.

The Endorphins and Enkephalins

Only recently did biochemists uncover the existence of potent pituitary proteins and peptides such as the *endorphins* and the *enkephalins* which can induce a state of pleasure in a body and which are produced by the body as a result of experiencing positive emotions. This appears to be one important link between a patient's *expectations* of health from a placebo and the biochemical changes which actually bring it about in the body. Not only do these neurotransmitters appear to serve as channels of communication within the brain and central nervous system, they also seem to link states of human consciousness with biochemical processes. For instance, some activate immune responses and help protect you from illness. Others can enhance learning ability, still others have remarkable anti-depressant activity or mediate such functions as sleep, breathing, heart-rate. And, although research into the exact channels by which your psychological state affects health is still searching for answers, the fact that it does is something you can make use of now. Meditation increases endorphin levels. Endorphins are also at least in part responsible for the feelings of 'high' which come when you exercise long and hard and they appear to be central to the human sexual response. Their production in the body is probably an important factor in creating high-level wellness and emotional wellbeing.

Developing an Ultrahealth Mindstyle.

Your imagination is one of the most potent tools for change you will find anywhere. Whether or not you are aware of it you use it all the time. You have a set of mind images about yourself which are clear and strong, and which operate for better or worse on your health, your relationships, your work, your abilities and your accomplishments. Most of these are unconscious. And, alas, for most people, many of them are negative; things like 'I'm always tired', 'I look old', 'I'm afraid of getting cancer', 'I could never succeed at that'. The variations on negativity are endless – but they have something in common: all such notions tend to lead you further away rather than closer to your goals of wellness, happiness and full functioning.

In fact, the situation is a lot more complex than this. For most of us tend to live on at least two levels at once. We have positive images of ourselves full of energy, young, good-looking, and successful which we allow to play through our minds. (It is often this particularly attractive persona which we try to display to the world.) Underneath however, if we are honest with ourselves, we are also plagued by doubts, inadequacies, a fear of failure and perhaps a sense of personal impotence or hopelessness. The latter comes from a fundamental assumption that a human being is basically powerless to change anything and that we are really only pawns in the game of life. Making effective use of your mind power to bring these two levels together, to soften a lot of the nagging self-doubts and strengthen your ability to make use of the imagination of whatever positive changes you want to achieve will put you leagues ahead in the play for ultrahealth. And the tools for doing this are really very simple – no weird psychic or airy-fairy practices. They are based on creating strong images in your mind of what the ultrahealth state is going to be like for *you*. It is, literally, the power of positive thinking.

Let your mind play on these images, rather like daydreams, whenever you're relaxing, exercising or simply stuck in commuter traffic – in other words, as often as you can. The stronger and clearer your positive images are, and the more detailed and personalized, the more useful they will be in becoming part of the everyday reality of your life. This, coupled with the clearly visible results of changes in your diet, regular aerobic exercise and all of the other tools that help you play the ultrahealth game will soon have you aware of just how very much personal power and autonomy you have. It is up to you to choose the way you want your life to be and then to make it that way.

Create an Ultrahealth Image for Yourself

Start now to dream of what it will be like for you to be ultrahealthy so you develop a number of clear mental pictures of yourself fit, well and looking great. But don't just consider the physical changes you would like to make. The optimally healthy person is a fully-functioning person – one who can make full use of his or her potential for fun and creativity as well. Get to know him or her and begin to see yourself in this image. Here are some of his or her characteristics:

- *An exceptional ability to cope with change and to learn from it.* Most people have trouble with change. It is unsettling and frightening. It needn't be. It all depends on how you look at it. An optimally healthy person will tend to view change not as threatening but as a challenge to learn from and grow from, whether the change at face value appears to be 'good' or 'bad'. And as far as failure is concerned, instead of being a source of fear for him, when he experiences it he views it as something that shows him how to deal with a similar situation in the future. He suffers no great sense of shame over making mistakes. After all, human beings *do* fail sometimes. He also functions particularly well under stress since he is free to deal with the tasks at hand instead of having to expend energy, boosting his own self-esteem or defending himself from possible failure.

- *No great worry about saying 'No'.* Assertiveness, not aggression, plays a central role in high-level health. It implies a strong sense of your individual right to your values and opinions and a tendency to respect the rights of other people as well. Developing healthy assertiveness can be quite a challenge for some people, particularly women who have been raised to believe they should always be 'nice' or to go along with whatever is asked of them. You need to be able to say no to a food or drink you don't really want, a request from a lover or spouse, a demand from a child or a colleague. The best way to develop healthy assertiveness is simply to practise it. It feels a bit strange at first but the more you do the easier it becomes. Then you avoid all the bad feelings and self-denial which go with too much 'niceness'. And paradoxically only when you are positively assertive can you discover what real unselfishness is, because then what you give is what you *choose* to give, not what you feel *obliged* to give. It is given freely with no strings attached.

- *A tolerance for ambiguity and a sense of balance.* When the kind of lifestyle you have chosen is one for ultrahealth, a certain expansiveness is created in which you can strive for the full use of your talents and express your creative impulses as fully as possible even in complex situations such as those where individual rights seem to come into conflict. You also create a sense of balance in judgement so that you can look at something and decide if it is of value to you quite apart from what the 'accepted' attitude to it may be. You tend not to go to extremes. You don't need them. If ever you do choose what appears to others to be an eccentric path, you do so without fanaticism, calmly, knowing simply that what you do appears at that moment with all the information you have to be best for *you*. You allow other people a lot of space to choose something completely different and respect their choices.

- *A well-conditioned body.* This not only brings you energy, it also helps you cope with stress better, look better and younger and strengthens your sense of self-reliance. Top-level fitness leads to a freedom to achieve excellence in other non-physical areas of your life as well. Being in top condition also makes it possible for you to work or play (or both) for long hours after you would have given out before. It increases stamina, strength and flexibility not only physically but emotionally as well.

- *A personal commitment to excellence.* This is reinforced constantly by how and what you eat, the physical and creative activities you choose to follow and the way you think about yourself and your life. Success is a thing a lot of people fear, although they are usually unaware of it. But succeeding can become an ordinary experience after making a few changes in your life habits. It is possible to strive for excellence without great effort and to live at a pace which allows you time to be successful and to enjoy it rather than having to grit your teeth and aim for something 'over there' which you feel secretly you may never achieve. The optimally healthy person chooses to make full use of his potentials and is not willing to settle for mediocrity. It just isn't good enough or interesting enough. There are hundreds of daily experiences which can become expressions of a commitment to excellence and wellbeing. Enjoy them.

- *A marked absence of common minor ailments and troubles.* Most people believe that the Monday morning 'blues' or the aches and pains in joints after forty are a normal part of living. But they take up little space in the life of the ultrahealth player. 'Normal' to him or her means moving with ease, and feeling pretty good about things day after day – sometimes feeling very good indeed – not because something stupendous has just happened but because when you are really fit and well that is the *normal* way to feel.

- *A sense that friendship is valuable and a concern for the needs of others.* Time invested in friendship with other people, in relation to animals, in a family and at work creates the kind of environmental support system that makes it easy for you to sustain disappointments, and, most important of all, to feel part of the human community. This sense of being an individual yet part of a greater whole is one of the most important foundations on which an ultrahealth lifestyle can be built. As a number of interesting studies show, it helps prevent illness as well. Pets matter too. They have been shown to mediate delinquent and destructive behaviour and they can even bring about healthy physical changes in the people who own them, such as lowering blood pressure that is too high.

- *Ageing is an individual matter.* We are all going to age – but how you do it is up to you. There is absolutely no reason to expect ageing to entail a loss of sexual potency, mental power or physical attractiveness. By learning the tools for counteracting premature or pathological ageing and making use of them, you can avoid both. By looking upon the whole process of getting older not as an inevitable decline but as a path towards wholeness it can become an exciting journey rather than an object of fear and loathing. You will also avoid the 'jazzy youth syndrome' which a lot of people over 40 suffer from, in which they tend to undermine their dignity by pretending to be younger than they are and feel apologetic for their maturity. Maturity is a blessing. Use it wisely, be proud of it.

- *Laughter comes easily.* An ability to laugh at the absurd (including yourself when appropriate) and a sense of fun are perhaps the most important of all the ultrahealth characteristics. Joy is health-giving. It is also an excellent anti-ageing device not only for the sense of youthful freedom it can bring but because of the specific biochemical changes in your body a hearty laugh brings about. Paradoxically, often the most delightful sense of humour parallels a strong sense of purpose in a person – another ultrahealth characteristic. People with a sense of meaning about their life are far freer to indulge their humour and experience their joy. And just as illness can be contagious, so can laughter. It may be the best gift you can give anybody.

- *A strong sense of self-esteem and a cheerful outlook.* You respect who you are. And you are free to be who you are, not forced to conform to some outer set of rules and regulations. Neither do you have to be superhuman to feel good about yourself. And when you come up against troubles or challenges your sense of self-importance is not laid on the line. Unlike most people, you don't sense yourself as helpless. Basically your self-image is alive and well and you have no great need to defend it. It is easy for you to feel humble yet proud in a positive way all at once. They are not necessarily mutually exclusive. Looking towards the future with such a self-image can be an exciting and expansive way to live. What lies ahead looks mysteriously interesting rather than fearful.

- *Integrity.* You set your own standards and you live up to them. Your values become a source of strength and energy for you. You don't have to compromise them to achieve some temporary advantage.

- *A vision of your place within the whole.* Optimally healthy people have a good sense of their relationship to the earth and to nature and feel responsibility towards their environment. This kind of ecological consciousness which encompasses not only self-respect but respect of what is 'other' is part of a world view implicit in ultrahealth. It is a world view that (unlike that based on Cartesian dualism which emphasizes the division between mind and matter, subject and object) emphasizes man's inter-relatedness with the earth. It views the individual as a psycho-biological unit – a total being whose thoughts and feelings and perceptions are intimately connected with his biochemistry and his physiology. And it views the healthy person as one whose whole system – both mind and body – is in a state of dynamic equilibrium not only within itself but in relation to the rhythms of the life around him or her. In such a state your health-promoting and restorative or healing functions are far stronger than the pathogenic or destructive ones. Moving towards ultrahealth is the process by which these good equilibriums are restored. The tools to help you do this – from vitamins to jogging – are of no particular value in their own right. They are only 'helpers' in the process of achieving ultrahealth.

Individualizing your Vision

Not all of these characteristics will appeal to everyone although they do tend to be pretty universal amongst the healthy people whose lives 'work' – what psychologist Abraham Maslow called the *self-actualizing* people, or Carl Rogers the *fully-functioning* people. Any which don't seem relevant to you, forget – for the moment. They might grow to be important as you get more involved in the ultrahealth game. If not, it doesn't matter. Those that do seem to have meaning, take a closer look at. Maybe make a few notes about them. How much do they apply to you, say on a scale of ten? Then look again in a few weeks. What may surprise you is that these things tend to become more characteristic of someone the more he or she follows a way of eating for high-level energy and makes use of all the other tools for ultrahealth. Refer to them often if you can. Keep them in mind and identify with them as much as possible. Set your imagination to work. This will not only make change for high-level wellness easier, it will clear away a lot of the old negative mental debris that may be weighing you down. In addition to the characteristics listed, add your own. Then, when you are relaxing or having a bath or working or whatever, let your mind play upon some of these things. They give a powerful boost to energy and wellness.

When in Doubt, Act 'As If'

There is a lot of power in the above suggestion. Pretence, which many people look askance at and demean, is often the mother of genuine improvement. The dilettante whose main interest in painting comes from a desire to impress at parties can find one day, wandering through the National Gallery that, caught unawares between silly statements about the pictures before him, he has been stung by the bee of real aesthetic experience. Many a genuine passion has begun with such pretence (or pretension!) and turned into something life-transforming for the pretender in the end. So it can be with ultrahealth. By 'pretending' to be as strong, healthy, energetic and self-aware as you would like to be, you both raise your expectations and put yourself in the frame of mind helpful to bring these things about. It's another trick that's helpful in ultrahealth play.

14
Techniques for Transformation

What About Other Mind Tools?
THE NUMBER OF techniques available in the west for expanding consciousness and altering attitudes from positive to negative is legion. They range from management training and sales promotion mind games through various forms of yoga and mind development, to Buddhist tantra. I have certainly not tried them all, but I know a number of people who claim benefit from practising various methods. From those which I do know well, I believe there are two techniques which stand out as particularly helpful in the search for ultrahealth. One is autogenic training – probably the simplest technique for dealing with stress ever developed in the west and one which has profound implications for mental and spiritual as well as physical health. The other, the Alexander Technique, is a demanding and highly disciplined approach to health, personal autonomy and mental clarity which can be of use regardless of your age or physical condition. It's a process of physical re-education concerned with changing the way you use your body as a whole.

Let's Look at Autogenic Training First
A thoroughly comprehensive and highly successful deep relaxation technique first presented in its entirety in 1932 by the German psychiatrist Johannes H. Schultz, autogenic training (AT) consists of a series of simple mental exercises designed to turn off the stress mechanisms in the body and turn on the restorative rhythms associated with profound psychophysical relaxation. It is a method which, when used daily, brings results comparable to those achieved by eastern meditators who have been working at their

practices for a long time. It is particularly appealing to the western mind because, unlike many forms of meditation and yoga, it has no cultural, religious or cosmological overtones and it requires no special clothing or unusual postures or rituals. One of the things which appeals most about it to me is, as the name implies, it is generated from *within*. The person practising AT has no external values or philosophies imposed upon him or her. But the implications of using AT go far beyond merely dealing with stress. It has proven itself to be a potent technique both for restoring health to unwell people, enhancing it in the well and expanding consciousness and heightening creativity in whoever uses it.

Control Over the Autonomic Nervous System

Schultz was a student of the clinically-orientated neuropathologist Oskar Vogt, who worked at the turn of the century at the Berlin Neurobiological Institute and was deeply involved in research on sleep and hypnosis. Vogt remarked that some of his patients who had been subjected to conventional forms of hypnosis soon developed the ability to put themselves in and out of a hypnotic state (or rather auto-hypnotic, since it was self-induced). He noticed that these patients experienced remarkable relief from tension and fatigue and also tended to lose whatever psychosomatic disorders they had been suffering from. Schultz drew on Vogt's observations and went on to design techniques for individuals to be able to induce this deep mental and psychological relaxation at will.

Schultz noticed that people entering the auto-hypnotic state experienced two specific physical phenomena: the first was a sensation of heaviness in their limbs and torso, and the second a feeling of diffuse warmth throughout the body. The feeling of warmth is the result of vasodilation in the peripheral arteries, and the sensation of heaviness is caused by deep relaxation in the body's muscles. Schultz thought that if he taught people to make suggestions to themselves that these things were happening to their bodies he could rapidly and simply introduce them to the state of 'passive concentration' which characterizes the auto-hypnotic state and can be used to exercise great influence over the autonomic nervous system to restore imbalance which prolonged stress has brought about.

Since most people tend to get 'stuck' in the sympathetic-dominated stressed state, gradually symptoms of anxiety, depression, insomnia and strain appear, and sometimes more serious stress-related conditions such as coronary disease, high blood pressure, ulcers, migraine and exhaustion develop. What Schultz found in his studies was that his patients were rapidly developing a capacity to switch from the sympathetic- to the parasympathetic-dominated state, so that they no longer remained trapped in stress. But when patients started to practise the simple technique he'd developed, some other rather exciting things began to happen too. Not only did they find they were able to deal with current stress levels easily, in a way which was difficult to describe, they also appeared to eliminate 'old' stress which had 'accumulated' in their body. With this came improved mental and bodily functioning plus apparently automatic elimination of maladaptive behaviour, as well as whatever neurotic or psychosomatic symptoms accompanied it.

The Oriental Paradox of Self-Induced Passivity

It was quite a discovery. The European scientific community found it hard to believe that something so simple could have such a profound effect. The early researchers had uncovered the fact that in this state of 'passive concentration' the activities governed by your autonomic nervous system can be influenced and rebalanced automatically – not through your exercising any conscious act of *will* but rather by learning to abandon yourself to an ongoing organismic process.

This strange paradox of self-induced passivity is central to the working of AT. It is also an important part of any ultrahealth lifestyle. It closely parallels the so-called passive volition of biofeedback training and meditation. It is a skill which eastern yogis, famous for their ability to resist cold and heat, to change the rate of their heartbeat, levitate and perform many other extraordinary feats, have long practised. But until the development of biofeedback and AT and the arrival of eastern meditation techniques, this passive concentration largely remained a curiosity in the west, where active, logical, linear, verbal thinking is encouraged to the detriment of the innate abilities to simply experience. In fact, many psychologists and physicians working in the field of stress studies and stress control believe that it is over-emphasis on the use of the conscious will in the west, on our *control*, that makes us so prone to stress-based illnesses in the first place.

Sensations of Heaviness and Warmth

To help patients induce the autogenic state, Schultz worked first with the sensations of heaviness and warmth and then added suggestions about regularity of heartbeat and gentle, quiet breathing – two more natural physiological characteristics of relaxation. He then went on to the sensation of abdominal warmth and coolness in the forehead. These six physiologically oriented directions – heaviness and warmth in the legs and arms, regulation of the heartbeat and breathing, abdominal warmth and cooling of the forehead – became the core of autogenic training and are known as the Autogenic Standard Exercises. The person practising AT goes through each of the six steps, one by one: 'My arms and legs are heavy and warm, my heartbeat is calm and regular etc.' each time he practises. Because of the body's and mind's ability with repetition to slip more and more rapidly into the deeply relaxed but highly aware AT state, the formula becomes increasingly shortened until, after a few weeks or months of practising three times a day, you can quickly induce a state of profound psycho-physical relaxation at will. And once the exercises have been mastered you can practise anywhere – even sitting on a bus.

The benefits of being able to do this are innumerable, some of them instant – such as counteracting acute stress or fatigue, refreshing yourself mentally and physically and clearing your mind for better thinking – others are long term. Patients with high blood pressure experience drops of from 11 to over 25 per cent in systolic blood pressure, as well as a 5 to 15 per cent diminution in diastolic pressure. Brainwave activity changes so that there is a better balance of right and left hemispheres, leading to improved creativity at work and in relationships and a better sense of being at peace with oneself. Recoveries from bronchial asthma and a whole range of other psychosomatic disorders have been reported, as well as highly successful 'spontaneous' modification of self-destructive behaviour patterns and habits such as drug-taking, compulsive eating and alcoholism.

How Is It Done?

The basic AT exercises are simple. Taking up one of three optional postures – sitting slumped rather like a rag doll on a stool, lounging in an easy chair, or lying on your back with your arms at your side –

you make sure you are reasonably protected from noise and disturbances and that your clothes are loose and comfortable. You close your eyes and focus your attention on your arms, one at a time, with the suggestion 'arms are heavy' several times. Then go on to 'legs are heavy', then 'arms and legs are warm', and so on, working through the six steps. As the exercise gets familiar it is simplified and instead of having to go through each limb separately, the suggestion 'my right arm is heavy' will trigger the psychophysical relaxation process in the whole body. (Some people get feelings of heaviness and warmth immediately, for others it takes as long as a week or two of practising three times a day for 10 or 15 minutes at a time. But for everyone it comes eventually and with it a profound sense of relaxation.) At the end of the series of self-directed instructions, you 'cancel' the training session by clenching your hands into fists and drawing them briskly to your shoulders, taking a deep breath, and then stretching. This brings about an immediate return to normal consciousness, although the temporary excursion into the realm of deep relaxation which you have just experienced will continue to exercise its benefits.

The reason this simple mental exercise should bring about such profound benefits is still at least a partial mystery. The neuro-physiological mechanism by which the autonomic nervous system is controlled is not completely understood. AT appears to bring about a state of passive concentration which lets your mind and body work towards more harmonious functioning. It appears to remove conflicting intention between cortical and sub-cortical processes so that you can achieve a higher level of psychosomatic wellbeing.

The Phenomenon of Autogenic Discharge

One of the most common questions asked about AT is how it differs from various eastern meditative techniques such as Transcendental Meditation and Zen. Although AT brings about a similar 'low arousal' state, where parasympathetic activity dominates, unlike classical meditation it stems from exercises meant specifically to induce simple physical sensations. These are intended to lead to a state of relaxation of a purely physical nature. But the experiences which accompany its practice are fascinating: in addition to slowing the heartbeat, reducing blood pressure and improving the depth of respiration, changes in the reticular activating system in the brain stem can, in a few people, bring about what are known as 'autogenic discharges'. These appear to be a spontaneous way of 'de-stressing' the body and eliminating old tensions. Autogenic discharges can manifest themselves as temporary twitching of the arms or legs (much like the twitch experienced occasionally on falling into a deep sleep) during the session itself, or increased peristaltic movement (stomach rumbles) or various transient emotions or feelings of dizziness or visual or auditory effects. These phenomena are completely harmless and usually quick to come and go and, according to autogenic practitioners, are an important part of throwing out life-accumulated disturbing material from the brain. Because of these effects it is sometimes recommended that AT is taught under medical supervision. In practice, they are rare, however, and most people can deal with them if and when they appear without difficulty.

Altered States of Consciousness

Once the initial basic training in AT has been mastered, you can go on to explore more subtle psychological aspects and to experience altered states of consciousness and develop a higher degree of autonomic control. For example, in the advanced stages of AT, participants have demonstrated abilities to anaesthetize themselves against third-degree burns, and to explore areas of symbolism and fantasy which can be useful in resolving internal dilemmas and conflicts. Numerous reports of self-healing have come from people who have gone on to explore advanced AT. And some experience breakthroughs of consciousness which parallel those achieved in advanced stages of eastern meditation. But whatever AT's more esoteric abilities, the most important of its virtues – for those intent on reaching a high level of wellness and preventing premature ageing – is the way in which, practised regularly, it not only makes it possible for you to deal with stress – while helping to prevent the development of stress-related illnesses – but creates high energy levels and a sense of wellbeing.

AT is a technique which, once you learn it, you can use for the rest of your life. By practising it even for a couple of minutes a day in a chair or even on a bus you can reap innumerable ultrahealth benefits. And, like the other super-helper, the Alexander Technique, it is a self-controlled method of awareness and change which seems to grow as you grow so that it never becomes redundant.

The Alexander Technique – Transformation Through the Body

Although it is often associated with fringe medicine, the Alexander Technique, which has been passed on from teacher to student for over 80 years, is quite different from treatments such as osteopathy and reflexology; neither is it some kind of posture training. It is a process of physical re-education concerned with changing the way you use your body as a whole; in doing this the entire mind-body relationship alters for the better. A course of training, consisting of half-hour sessions – first once or twice a week, and later once every few months, can last from a few months to a few years. The therapy itself is deceptively simple. It consists of little more than the very gentle handling of the head and neck and then the whole body – shoulders, chest, pelvis, legs and feet – to correct the way in which they are held and used when standing, walking, sitting and moving. Yet it is based on highly sophisticated observations on the part of the teacher and complex skills.

Towards Correct Usage

Using his or her hands and eyes the teacher continually monitors the student's body and readjusts his procedures, at the same time telling and showing the student how he has been using his body wrongly and helping him discover how it feels to use it correctly. But what is 'correct'? There is no rigid answer. Basically 'correct' is moving, standing and holding your body in the ways which work best so that you keep it free of pain and physical deformity – avoiding curved backs, hunched shoulders or peculiar walking habits.

The implications of using the body correctly can be far-reaching and lead to the improvement or cure of such apparently unrelated conditions as peptic ulcers, spastic colon, ulcerated colitis, eczema and rheumatoid arthritis as well as headaches caused by tension, asthma, low back pain and fibrositis. Students also report extra-ordinary changes in their emotional lives – the falling away of long-term anxiety and depression, a new sense of lightness and energy, and an unexpected sense of delight in using their body either for sports or simply moving about. Athletes and performers – from actors to violinists – claim the technique has brought them new dexterity and expressiveness in their work.

The Body as a Unified Organism

It is difficult for someone who has not experienced the Alexander Technique to imagine how simple alterations in the way the muscles are used can have profound implications for one's emotional and mental life. To a large extent this is because, thanks to the (often conscious) concept of mind-body dualism to which our civilization unfortunately adheres, we believe that mind and body are separate entities which have to be treated in isolation. The doctor heals the body with drugs, leaving the mind to the psychotherapist or psychoanalyst.

The precepts on which the Alexander Technique is based are quite different. Far ahead of his time, F. Matthias Alexander presented a view of the body as a unified organism. He saw man as a whole and viewed physical and psychological distortion as diseased states. He reasoned that the imbalances which showed themselves in misuse of the body could be corrected physically. When they were, the entire organism would function as it was meant to – mentally, physically and spiritually. How he came upon this notion and developed his technique is a story of unusual perceptiveness and persistence.

Born in Tasmania in 1869, Alexander had decided to become a 'reciter of dramatic and humorous pieces'. But before long he found that he had developed some serious voice difficulties which made his work as a performer virtually impossible. He sought medical help without success, and finally decided to try on his own to discover a remedy. He would stand for hours in front of the mirror and gradually came to realize that his voice was at its worst when he took the particular stances for reciting which felt 'right' to him. He continued to experiment with the use of his body's muscular system for several years until, after painstaking observation, readjustment and experiment directed at changing the way he used his body, he regained control of his voice.

The discovery of how badly he had been misusing his body led Alexander to observe that the majority of people in the western world stand, sit and move in an equally defective way – although they are usually totally unconscious of what they are doing wrong. With the support of an Australian doctor, he set out to teach what he had learned, first to actors, then to others.

Breaking the Chain of Determinism

Alexander believed that 'civilization' meant that man could no longer trust his instincts about what felt right for him and what did not, and that, if man was to survive and fulfil his potential, he would have to reintegrate his behaviour on a conscious level – through his body. The technique which he devised was a way of doing this. He also started to lecture and write about the technique. His success brought widespread recognition, fostered by some of his well-known students, such as the biologist George C. Coghill, William Jones and Aldous Huxley, who saw the method as a way of breaking the 'chains of determinism' and clearing the way for spiritual and physical experiences which had not been possible before.

It is perhaps surprising that the Alexander Technique has always tended to attract intellectuals, for it is very different in its approach from other types of educational training. Like autogenic training, it is not based on analytic concepts which divide mind from body by placing the achievements of goals above all else, as traditional western education tends to. Alexander called such an approach to learning 'end-gaining' and proposed instead a 'means-whereby' principle through which the student is shown how to inhibit his or her stereotyped responses, that is, the results of habit patterns and conditioning which are reflected in the ways he or she uses their body. This opens the way for a new conscious control and choice of direction. The inhibition of wrong use, in effect, makes possible the discovery of right use.

Head and Neck are Fundamental

In practical terms, Alexander training begins with work on the neck and head, for their misuse is regarded as fundamental: until this is corrected, misuse in the rest of the body cannot be put right. It is also here that most misuse starts. Dr. Wilfred Barlow, who with his wife had been largely responsible for carrying on the work of Alexander in Britain, described the base of the neck region as 'a veritable maelstrom of muscular coordination'. In this area, wrong patterns of breathing put muscles into excessive spasm, where the functions of speech and swallowing occur and the blood vessels and nerves pass through on their way to the brain.

Right use implies a dynamic balance between the weight of the head and the degree of tension in the muscles of the neck, so that the head acts as an inertial system which can be moved freely in any direction without any sensation of weight. According to Barlow, in 99 out of 100 people it does not. Instead, excessive and wrongly distributed muscle tension inhibits neck movement and can throw various bodily mechanisms – from breathing to the flow of blood to the brain – out of balance. For example, when most people go to sit down, instead of lowering themselves into the chair simply, they retract their head, shortening the muscles at the back of the neck. This simple, habitual reaction can not only result in a hump at the base of the neck but also in other distortions of the back and shoulders, pelvis and limbs to compensate for the primary misuse. And, most important of all, the postures which result have a profound effect on how a person feels about him- or herself, and relates to the world.

An Extraordinary Sense of Lightness

The Alexander teacher first makes his subject aware of the way he habitually pulls back his head and then helps him inhibit this automatic response. He is then able to release a set of reflexes which makes the student's new movements easier, freer and more pleasant, and eventually changes the whole relationship between the head and trunk region. As this happens, students report an extraordinary sense of lightness which affects all their movements and can last from a few minutes to several hours or even days. Students claim that you cannot imagine this feeling unless you have experienced it. The Alexander Technique teacher then works with the student to re-educate his use of muscles, not just in the neck area but all over the body, gradually bringing him an awareness of the difference between good use and misuse.

In recent years many well-known writers, artists, musicians and scientists have sung the praises of the Alexander Technique. Nobel laureate Nicholas Tinbergen, Professor of Animal Behaviour at Oxford, devoted half his acceptance speech to it. Impressed by what Alexander had achieved in terms of relief of human suffering, yet sceptical of the many claims for the technique, Tinbergen had decided to undergo the training himself with his wife and daughter. Between them, they soon noticed 'striking improvements in such diverse things as high blood pressure, breathing, depth of sleep, overall cheerfulness and mental alertness, resilience to outside pressures and also in such a refined skill as playing a stringed musical instrument'. One of the things about the technique which most seemed to impress Tinbergen was that it could be effective in someone who had already subjected himself to 40 to 50 years of steady misuse.

The Alexander Technique has come to the attention of many of the new wave psychologists as well. They believe that the learning process is a physical matter, not just something that takes place in the splendid isolation of the brain. They also believe that it is profoundly related, quite literally, to how one stands. For instance, ingrained diffidence has both physical and psychological consequences. Working with the Alexander Technique cannot undo all the negative socialization people accrue, but it can make a significant dent in it. It also brings about profound changes both in your appearance, your health and your view of yourself – even in your view of the world.

PART FIVE

AGELESS AGEING

15
The Kronos Challenge

AS AN ULTRAHEALTH player, the most insidious foe you will ever have to pit your wits against is Kronos – the god of time. There appears to be no way to destroy what Milton called his 'silent touches'. We can, however, go a long way towards softening them. As science probes the secrets of the cell and begins to decipher the genetic code, theories about slowing down the process of ageing are rapidly turning into practical techniques for doing so. Researchers have already been able to do this for animals and in some cases even to reverse age-related changes. Now they can also double an animal's lifespan. The pattern of age changes in humans appears to be very similar to those of the animals they are working with.

The Three Faces of Ageing

There are almost as many theories as to what ageing is all about as there are scientists studying the process. Generally speaking, however, research falls into three main areas about which there is much agreement: 'genetic clocks', random damage and the immune system. First, there seems to be some kind of internal genetic 'clock' or 'clocks', the control for which is probably centred in the cells themselves or an area of the brain, that appears to 'switch off' specific vital functions at certain times. This could account for a number of 'life events' which tend to occur around the same period in almost everyone, such as the way women go through menopause. Just where and what these age clocks in the body might be is still debatable. Once we learn what they are, and how to manipulate or to reset them, we should be able to reprogramme predetermined occurrences so that our bodies age much more slowly. But there is, as yet, very little in the way of practical treatments or advice from age-researchers on how to do this.

The second major area of age-research and practical methods designed to slow ageing lies in the process of cumulative wear and tear your body goes through – the kind of random damage on a cellular level which is triggered by external agents such as ultraviolet light, air pollution, poisons in food or in the environment, alcohol, tobacco, drugs – simply the by-products of metabolism in the body. These influences result in the formation of *free radicals* – highly reactive molecules which do serious damage to the body. Alex Comfort once referred to these free radicals as 'promiscuous' because, 'like delegates at a conference, they seem to race around frantically combining with everything'. They are a major cause of *cross-linking* which makes your body's protein tissues age rapidly and results in wrinkled skin, stiff limbs and a degenerating cardiovascular system. About combating age-related changes in this area there is much information and even a number of practical suggestions as to what you can do now.

The All-Important Immune System

Central to the whole question of ageing is the third area of intensive research which investigates the role that a gradually weakening immune system plays in ageing. As you get older your immune system, which is responsible for protecting your body against invasion, illness and allergy, gradually loses these capacities. Its functions decline and your body becomes more susceptible to illness, bacterial invasions and deterioration. A poorly functioning immune system is also much more likely to attack your body's own cells in error. This produces what are known as 'auto-immune' disorders such as arthritis. When your body is not able to repair random damage done by wear and tear, you get into a kind of vicious circle of age decline where the immune system is further weakened. In turn, it is less able to protect your body from further random damage. A lot of people have come to believe that this downward spiral is an inevitable part of growing older. But is it? There are a number of very good treatments which appear to offer support to the immune system and prolong its potency. Some may even help prevent ageing and repair random damage at the same time. They can play an important part in any well-informed bid to keep Kronos in his place. Remember that editorial in the journal of the American Medical Association which said we are supposed to 'die young in old age, but free from disease'? That should be the ultrahealth player's attitude to ageing. You can look and feel great at 60 or even 70 and beyond; you need never lose brain power as the years pass. Time doesn't *have* to take its toll.

How Old Are You?

Not an easy question to answer. For, regardless of when you were born, you are at least *three* ages: your chronological age as measured by the calendar, your psychological age and your biological age – probably the most important of all. In fact, the latest research into ageing indicates that the rate at which you age has but little to do with the simple passage of time. There are far too many other variables, like genetic inheritance, the food you eat, the way you live, your mental attitude and the number of pollutants in your environment – to name only a few. The ultrahealth lifestyle outlined so far can have an all-encompassing effect on holding back the ageing process all by itself – simply because the things you do to achieve a state of high-level wellness and vitality just happen to be the things which many age-researchers insist are important in slowing down body degeneration. But, some insist, there are a number of other things you can do as well. The most important of all – one which has now been conclusively proven in many animal experiments, and about which there is no controversy – is *eat less*. Weight does add years!

Secrets of the Long-Lived

Dr. Alexander Leaf, from Harvard Medical School, spent several years studying three cultures where the people were exceptionally long-lived (some claimed to be as old as 140), but who at the same time showed few signs of degenerative changes traditionally associated with age. They were the Vilcabamba Indians in an Andes valley, the Hunzas in a mountainous part of Kashmir, and the Abkhazians in (former) Soviet Georgia. They suffered neither tooth decay, heart disease, mental illness, obesity nor cancer. Leaf wanted to find out what these peoples had in common and to discover the secrets behind their youth. He discovered that they led extremely active lives, regardless of their age, and that they had vigorous sex lives well into their eighties and nineties. Men and women of ninety or more also spent many hours each day in physical labour – for physical fitness was an inevitable consequence of the active life of these peoples. They also ate a very low-calorie diet. While the average Briton or American eats somewhere between 3,000 and 3,500 calories a day, his Vilcabamban brother contents himself with a mere 1,700. Also, in all three groups, their diet – like the ultrahealth diet – was low in fats and in proteins from animal sources and high in fresh foods, a great many of them eaten raw. All of their foods were grown organically as these people had no access to artificial fertilizers. They had never heard of sugar but ate mostly rough grains, fresh vegetables and fruits.

Eat Less and Stay Young

Over 50 years ago a researcher at Cornell University, Clive McCay, noticed that brook trout which were growth-retarded as a result of being underfed lived far longer than normal-sized trout. He experimented with rats to see what effect feeding them on a very low-calorie diet from birth would have on their lifespan. He found that these animals on a calorie-deprived diet – which was carefully supplemented with nutrients so the rats did not suffer deficiencies – had increased lifespans. This was by far and away the most exciting practical discovery anybody had made in the area of how to make an animal live longer. But it was relatively useless to human beings since nobody would attempt to restrict a baby's diet in the same way from birth, because of the possible risk of brain damage. Also restricted animals are smaller than fully-fed ones and a small percentage of the restricted group tends to die very young. So for many years McCay's findings were largely ignored by those looking for concrete anti-ageing methods.

Recently however a number of studies in the United States and Australia have concentrated on the effect of calorie restriction on lifespan of 'middle-aged' animals – studies not begun on the animals until, in human terms, they are in their forties. One of the scientists who has done much in this area is Roy Walford, a professor at the University of California Medical School and one of the world's leading experts on ageing. In projects which Walford describes as 'undernutrition without malnutrition' – administering a diet low in calories but high in basic nutrients such as vitamins and minerals – he has been able to add 40 per cent to the maximum lifespan of mice and keep fish alive 300 per cent longer than usual.

Underfeeding Improves Immune Responses

The exact mechanisms by which dietary restriction extends life is still largely a mystery. But researchers do know that a low-calorie but nutritionally potent diet substantially improves immune system functioning – in effect, by rejuvenating it – so that signs of auto-immune responses are markedly reduced. It seems also to protect the immune system from the usual age-degeneration an animal is subjected to so that its ability to combat disease and eliminate toxic materials from the body, which ordinarily declines to a level of 10 or 20 per cent of what it was in youth, occurs only very slowly. Instead, the immune response of these highly nourished but underfed animals remains excellent. Their bodies, unlike those of 'normal' ageing animals, are able to repair much of the age-related damage that occurs at a cellular level and are prevented from turning against themselves.

Restricted animals also show increased intelligence and have a much lower incidence of degenerative illness such as cancer and heart disease. What disease does occur comes only much later in the animal's life. And how great a calorie restriction appears necessary to bring about these beneficial changes? The diet of Walford's mice had been restricted by about a third of the calories they were raised on.

Walford's work and the work of other scientists using calorie restriction has generated a great deal of excitement about what human beings might do now to lengthen lifespan and to avoid age-degeneration. Many age-experts have begun to recommend that healthy people who have already attained their full growth and maturity could benefit from restricting their calories to somewhere between 1,500 and 2,000 calories a day (depending on how active a life you lead). But cutting down on calories is only half the formula. It just won't do to go on some slimming regime you find in a magazine, you need high-potency nutrition with it. Processed foods play no part in any such diet. The foods that you do eat have to be superbly high in nutritional value – fresh fruits and vegetables (as many as possible eaten raw), wholegrain cereals and breads, pulses and seeds with very little fat and only moderate protein (see page

102). Your food intake has to be balanced and no salt should be added to foods – salt is something which in animal studies has been shown to shorten lifespan considerably. Such a diet is, by its very nature, also high in fibre. Most experts also insist that you supplement your diet with a full complement of essential vitamins and minerals.

Is Ageing All in the Mind?

Perhaps more than you might think. Psychologists have found that many of the changes that take place in our bodies and minds associated with ageing depend on our 'programmed expectations'. In our society it is assumed for instance that at thirty the first wrinkles appear, at forty 'middle-aged spread' sets in, and at seventy the mind begins to lose its clarity. But according to studies only 12 per cent of the population has even the slightest pre- disposition to the kind of changes that result in senility; yet as people get older they become increasingly worried about it until they may work themselves into a kind of vicious circle of depression and anxiety which results in decline. How you age may have a lot to do with what you *expect* to happen. Change your expectations and that can change too.

Regular Fasts Can Help Too

Periodic fasting of animals is another way of restricting calories which has shown itself to be useful in increasing their lifespan. This is a fact which I find particularly interesting because European experts on fasting have for a hundred years been saying that done sensibly and regularly for short periods and in combination with a nutritionally excellent diet, fasting will make you live longer and reduce the incidence of illnesses.

Roy Walford tends to be slightly more liberal with his own calories than sticking to a rigid 1,500 a day. But he then fasts for two days a week in order to end the week with the recommended number of calories. He claims that a healthy normal-weight adult will lose weight on such a regime but only very slowly until you have lost, say, about one fourth to one fifth of the weight you were when you started. Such weight-loss appears to have no disadvantages (unless you fancy yourself slightly plump for aesthetic reasons) and indeed may be an important factor in the way such a calorically restricted, but nutritionally superb, regime appears to improve immune functions. And because the weight-loss is so slow – it occurs in normal-weight people at a rate of, perhaps, six pounds a year until they reach their 'plateau' at which they remain – there is no chance of becoming flabby or tired from it. Indeed, such a regime tends to create the most extraordinary amounts of energy, according to people following it.

Raw Power For Youth

A diet high in raw foods (where they make up 75 per cent of the calories you eat) has quite remarkable rejuvenating abilities. It raises the microelectric potentials of the cells, increases oxygenation and eliminates stored wastes and toxins which interfere with proper cell metabolism and cause cross-linking. It will also keep you mentally alert, make you lose excess weight and it tends to eliminate feelings of depression associated with ageing.

Regular Exercise Keeps You Fit

Your body was made for use. When you regularly pursue an aerobic form of exercise, you help to protect your cardiovascular system from arteriosclerosis (which is otherwise inevitable) and you increase your metabolic rate, which helps protect against fat – a precursor to many degenerative diseases. Exercise also protects you from disturbances in blood-sugar such as adult-onset diabetes and from high blood pressure, and relieves many mental conditions often associated with age such as depression. Aerobic exercise improves circulation and optimal oxygenation of the tissues in your body – one of the most important measurements for health and vitality.

Exercise Makes You Look Younger

As far as good looks are concerned this increased circulation brings to your skin cells a better supply of the nutrients needed for their proper functioning. It also more efficiently carries away wastes which can contribute to genetic damage in your cells and to cross-linking of the collagen which produces wrinkles. Albert Kligman, one of America's leading dermatologists, believes that exercise may serve another purpose in retarding skin ageing as well: if you keep yourself really fit you may lay down more fibrous proteins in the dermis, that deep layer of the skin where the structural network of *collagen* and *elastin* fibres gives strong young skin its firmness and cushiony feel. Then your face will preserve its youthful contours.

Another way in which vigorous exercise helps to hold back skin ageing is connected with the relationship between muscle and hormone production in the body. The amount of physical activity you get is a significant factor in maintaining optimal functioning of endocrine glands which provide hormones that are not only vital to youth and energy, but keep the skin smooth and soft in appearance. When you don't work out regularly, muscle mass declines. So does the amount of steroid hormones from the adrenals and sex glands – in direct proportion to the decrease in muscle mass, not (as was once believed) simply as a result of the ageing process itself. Rebounding, swimming, dancing or running for 30 minutes or more several times a week can prevent these degenerative musculo-skeletal changes from happening and help you maintain optimal levels of hormones essential to skin softness and resiliency. When you are inactive, even for as little as 24 hours, your muscle mass starts to deteriorate.

The Exercise-Age Controversy

Lounge-lizards are forever congratulating themselves on the fact that they don't 'waste their time' exercising. They cite well-known studies which are purported to show that exercise will make you die younger. It's a great excuse. The trouble is that when you examine some of the research they refer to you find that it is all based on the popular method of examining death records of athletes – a method which is faulty in a number of ways. For instance, there was a study carried out at Michigan State University comparing 629 varsity athletes with 583 non-athletes which showed that there was no difference in life length. Another at Harvard involving some 6,300 athletes showed that they died significantly *earlier* than the non-athletes. Their definition of the athlete was someone who was active athletically while at university. But the problem is that just because a man plays football or runs during his university career does not mean that he continues to exercise afterwards. Most athletes give up their training once they leave the atmosphere of the university. This was demonstrated by an interesting study carried out at University of Auckland in New Zealand. Looking at the training habits of 100 athletes out of season, Michael Colgan and his team of researchers found that only 34 of them continued training once the season finished. Studies examining the death records of former university athletes are of no use in determining what effect regular exercise has on lifespan.

The only studies that are able to assess the effect of training on ageing are those which attempt to measure how active a person is *throughout* his life, such as the one published in 1977 by Charles Rose and Michael Cohen from the Veterans Administration Hospital in Boston. With the help of relatives who were able to rate their level of physical activity from sedentary to very active, researchers – using the death records of 500 men – discovered that men who continued throughout their life to exercise in their leisure time lived 7.1 years longer than those whose level of activity had declined with the passing of the years. Other studies have shown that ordinary athletes who continue to exercise even as they grow old (up to 90 in some cases) show much less physical degeneration than non-athletes. They shrink in height only half as much, have a far better musculo-skeletal system, less body fat, and better heart and lung function.

Hydrochloric Acid and Ageing
A decline in hydrochloric acid in the stomach is a common event with the passing of the years. It results in an inability to break down proteins in your foods into their constituent amino acids so that the body can make use of them for rebuilding tissue and making enzymes and hormones. This can be remedied by taking food supplements of HCL and digestive enzymes with meals containing protein foods. This is especially true with *animal* protein foods.

Diet, Exercise and Rejuvenation
Not only can changing your diet to one more in line with ultrahealth principles – and getting yourself into a programme of regular aerobic exercise – help retard your own ageing rate and make you feel great, it can also rejuvenate your whole body, quite apart from whether or not you choose to make use of any of the other anti-ageing devices now available, from nutritional supplements to organic-specific antisera.

Your body is not the fixed size and shape you may believe it to be.

It changes slowly with use. And these changes can be for the better or for the worse. Most of your body's cells completely renew themselves so that the cells you have today are not the ones you will have five years from now. I have seen bodies and faces with flaccid muscles and loose skin be transformed in a few months by those two simple things, diet and exercise. They are far more powerful than any of the more sophisticated and more expensive rejuvenation treatments and really they will cost you nothing more than commitment and a little time.

16
The Mega Nutrient Approach

WHEN YOUR SKIN wrinkles, when rubber windscreen wipers harden and crack, and when the hide of an animal is turned into leather by the chemical process of tanning, what has taken place is cross-linking as a result of free radical damage. This is a phenomenon that occurs in the presence of oxygen and appears to be central to the ageing process in the whole body. In effect iron (which rusts), rubber (which cracks) and flesh (which wrinkles) all fall victim to the very molecule which brings us life: oxygen. Of course we could not live without oxygen. In the special energy factories of each muscle cell, called the mitochondria, we use it to burn fuel to give energy. But oxygen in the wrong place, or used in the wrong way, is inevitably involved in causing you to age fast. For instance, in the presence of certain chemicals in the body, or ultraviolet light, collagen fibres in the skin can oxidize and become cross-linked, rather than remaining in orderly rows. In this way they lose their pliancy and you form wrinkles.

In effect cross-linking is simply a process in which undesirable bonds are formed in the presence of oxygen. These chemical bonds can be between proteins (as in the case of crossed-linked collagen), lipids or nucleic acids which make up the cells' genetic material – the DNA and RNA. Some cross-linking is necessary in order to give your tissues strength and make them sturdy. But inappropriate cross-links which occur in the ageing process only increase the risk of cancer, arteriosclerosis and a number of other degenerative diseases such as arthritis. As one of the world's most famous age-researchers Johan Bjorksten, who formulated the cross-linking theory of ageing, says, 'many of these cross-linked molecules lead to agglomerates which cannot be broken down by any body enzyme, but will increase in the cell and gradually crowd out other constituents, thereby causing continued decline in the cell's activity and the ability to cope with stresses'. From an aesthetic point of view – how your skin looks – such a decline in cellular activity implies a slowing down of the reproductive process in the skin as well as the hardening and bunching together of the skin's supportive collagen which makes it prone to wrinkling and to sagging contours.

What Causes Cross-Linking?

There are a number of powerful cross-linkers which have been implicated in the ageing process in humans – chemicals or energy sources which increase the level of cross-linking and therefore the rate at which your body ages. They include ultraviolet light, acetaldehydes, ozone, ketones (which are found in the blood of diabetics and people on a high-protein, carbohydrate-free slimming regime), heavy metal ions such as aluminium, lead and cadmium, x-rays and free radicals (highly reactive atoms or molecules which can form toxic peroxides that damage and destroy cells). Many common environmental influences contain chemicals which belong to this list.

Acetaldehyde occurs both in cigarette smoke and as a common urban air pollutant. It is a potent cross-linker. So is the lead in petrol fumes, the aluminium which may be absorbed through regular use of some anti-perspirants, and cadmium, a build-up of which can occur in your body when you drink coffee regularly. Drinking alcohol spurs the production of acetaldehyde in your liver which can trigger further cross-linking, as can eating any kind of rancid oil or fat, since these react with radiation or form free radicals as a simple part of their metabolic breakdown in your body. Lying in the sun or on a tanning bed (no matter what kind of ultraviolet rays manufacturers tell you have been filtered out) may well be the single most dangerous practice of all for your skin. It damages the genetic materials of the skin cells, the collagen, and the lipids in the cell walls by causing them to undergo several types of free radical reactions including peroxidation and cross-linking.

Ageing and Oxygen Question

Oxygen plays an important positive part in protecting the body from age-related damage too. 'Maximum oxygen consumption' is the way scientists measure your body's ability to transport and make use of oxygen for cell metabolism. As you get older this ability decreases at the rate of about 1 per cent a year. The lower your oxygen consumption the less vitality you have and the more susceptible you are to many illnesses. An aerobic exercise programme followed regularly over a few weeks can recapture 40 years' worth of oxygen capacity which has been lost through a sedentary way of life.

Vitamin E supplements of 600–800 IU a day can increase the utilization of available oxygen by as much as 40 per cent.

Avoiding the Cross-Linkers

Before you even consider what kind of nutritional defence you might make use of to protect your body from the cross-linking process, start by eliminating as many of its known causes as you can from your life – like exposure to the sun when your body is unprotected by a sunscreen, cigarettes, drugs and alcohol. Then you are ready to consider how you can make use of what is known about the 'cures for the random damage free radicals and cross-linkers cause'.

Protection – the Second Line of Defence

It is almost impossible to live in a twentieth-century urban environment and avoid all these cross-linkers. So the second move in combating cellular ageing is to consider incorporating into your diet fairly large quantities of substances which have anti-oxidant properties – substances which have an ability to protect the body's genetic materials, proteins, from age-related damage.

A great deal of research done in the past 30 years (most of it with animals, for obvious ethical reasons) indicates that there are some very effective substances for doing this. According to many of the most respected age-researchers such as Bjorksten, Denham Harman, Al Tappel and others, eating properly and adding these substances to your diet can minimize the amount of free radical damage to your body. These 'age retarders' are often called anti-oxidants because they have ways of combating damaging oxidative reactions caused by radiation, chemicals and free radicals. Some are substances which occur naturally in our foods, although you would need to take them in much larger quantities to make use of their anti-ageing properties.

They include catechols which are found in bananas and potatoes, the phenolics – found in grapes – vitamins such as A, E, C and members of the B complex – especially B12, pantothenic acid, B6, and the bioflavonoids which occur in the white soft inner skin or pith of the peel of citrus fruits – as well as betacarotene and some amino acids such as cysteine (available in eggs), tyrosine and L-dopamine, plus the trace minerals zinc and selenium. Many age-researchers now recommend taking fairly high quantities of the vitamins, minerals, food substances and amino acid 'age retarders' as protection against free radical damage and cross-linking.

Stay Away from the Cross-Linkers

• **Don't smoke**. Stay away from people who do, particularly if you are in an enclosed area or small room. Not only does the acetaldehyde cross-link with collagen, the benzopropyrene (another chemical in cigarette smoke) depletes your system of vitamin C, making it unavailable for the production of new healthy collagen and encouraging it to wrinkle faster.

• **Stay out of the sun** unless your body is protected by a high-potency sunscreen which filters out *both* UVA and UVB rays. Never allow your face to tan at all. Protect it with a total block when you are in the sun. (There are some excellent after-shave tinted mois-turizers for men and gel makeups for women which give you the look of a healthy tan if you like without causing damage to skin – or harmless 'instant tan' lotions.)

• **Beware of unsaturated fats.** Not that your body doesn't need them, it does. But in small quantities only. Because polyunsaturates are so very unstable chemically, they easily become rancid (as do shell-less nuts which incidentally also contain polyunsaturates). And rancid or highly processed lipids are dangerous. The best oil to use for cooking is cold-pressed virgin olive oil, a monounsaturate which is remarkably stable. You can get other essential fatty acids from eating fish, shellfish, game, wholegrains, avocados, nuts and seeds.

• **Go easy on the alcohol.** Better yet, give it up altogether. Not only does it trigger acetaldehyde production in your liver, it depletes your body's supplies of some of the most important nutritional 'protectors' against free radical damage and cross-linking vitamins C and B1. Spirits are particularly damaging in this sense and are best avoided. As mentioned earlier, a glass of wine a day can aid digestion – but if you find you can't stop after a glass (and many people can't), then temperance is probably the best choice.

• **Check on heavy metals.** Consider having the presence of heavy metals in your body investigated. This can be done in a laboratory from a small sample of hair. An increasing number of doctors concerned with preventative care are using hair mineral analysis as a part of their diagnostic equipment. If high levels of heavy metals such as lead, aluminium, chromium, arsenic and so forth are found, they can be gradually removed from the system by careful use of specific nutritional substances such as vitamin C, pectin – a form of fibre which occurs in good quantity in apples – and garlic oil.

• **Banish Deodorants.** Avoid the use of anti-perspirants containing aluminium salts which are absorbed through the skin.

• **Give Up Drinking Coffee.** Besides causing a build-up of cadmium, the caffeine in coffee can cause other age-related changes.

Designing a Personalized Formula of Nutrients

This can be a complex business. For instance, some of the substances which are important can be dangerous if taken in too high a dosage. Chronic poisoning has been known to occur when vitamin A is taken in doses of 100,000 IU a day over several months. Selenium too can be poisonous if one gets too much of it. Vitamin E needs to be used with caution by anyone with a tendency to high blood pressure, beginning with low doses of 50 or 100 IU a day and only gradually increasing. And, of course, many of the vitamins and minerals have synergistic relationships which you should be aware of. For instance if you take a B vitamin individually, you must support it by a supplement containing the full B complex in order to avoid creating any deficiencies of other B vitamins over a long period of time. If you take a lot of vitamin E you will need less A, since E protects A from oxidizing so more is available for use in your body. Vitamin supplements should *help* – not harm – your health quotient.

Supplements to Fight Ageing

Studies on animals and some on humans show that certain nutrients can effectively combat ageing in two main ways:

• By preventing oxidation damage and cross-linking and perhaps by correcting part of the damage which has already occurred.

• By improving the functioning of the immune system.

But these nutrients have to work together to work best. For instance, selenium when taken in very small quantities together with large amounts of vitamin E and vitamin C creates a potent anti-oxidant force for use in the body. Used together these nutrients also enhance immune responses far more than they can when used separately.

Vitamin A and the Immune System

This vitamin is a particularly interesting 'age retarder', quite apart from its anti-oxidant properties. It is a powerful stimulant to the immune system – and a decline in the immune system, you'll remember, appears to be central to most age-related degeneration in the body. Vitamin A, or betacarotene which is a precursor to vitamin A, increases the size of the thymus gland – the directing centre of immune activity – and increases its functional capacity. Vitamin A has been shown to help protect against cancer, and to slow down the development of malignancy in epithelial cells where the disease is already present. It is also an excellent protector of skin, encouraging cell growth, stabilizing cell membranes and maintaining proper lubrication through adequate sebum production.

Vitamin C, Interferon and Homeostasis

Vitamin C, which counteracts many destructive chemicals in foods and our environment, also boosts the immune system so that your body can more efficiently ward off infection and sickness – including degenerative diseases such as cancer and vascular problems. In part this is because the vitamin stimulates the production of *interferon* – one of the body's natural anti-viral, anti-cancer chemicals. The vitamin has been shown to lower blood cholesterol in many people. In fact it appears to maintain physiological homeostasis (equilibrium) throughout the system. In the words of Irwin Stone, one of the world experts on vitamin C:

> On a molecular basis, the whole living process is nothing more than an orderly flow and transfer of electrons. Therefore, having an abundance of a substance like ascorbic acid present in living matter makes this orderly flow and transfer of electrons proceed with greater ease and facility. It acts substantially like an oil for the machinery of life.

Together with the trace element zinc, vitamin C plays a central role in the production of new collagen in your skin and throughout the body. It helps rebuild the protein in your skin that keeps it firm and resilient. The bioflavonoids (which occur in good quantity in citrus fruits and complement the action of vitamin C in the body) are also essential for strong, resilient collagen and for the maintenance of smooth, unlined skin. They help protect the integrity of tiny capillaries which, when they become fragile with age, tend to show up as 'spider veins' on cheeks and anywhere else the skin is particularly thin.

Vitamin E and Life-Extension

Vitamin E is the most important fat-soluble anti-oxidant found in nature. Experimentally, the lifespan of mice has been increased by 50 per cent by giving them supplements of it. Probably because it slows down cellular ageing due to random damage, it appears to be useful in holding back the appearance of telltale signs and symptoms of ageing.

Studies of animals deficient in the nutrient show striking similarities between a vitamin E deficiency and the characteristics of advanced age. Like vitamins A and C, it is also a stimulant to the immune system. A number of studies indicate it can be useful in warding off infection, heart attacks, and damage from air pollution as well as heightening your resistance to cancer.

These three vitamins, along with the other anti-oxidant nutrients are beginning to be formulated into nutritional supplements which people can take as they would an ordinary vitamin pill (although many prefer to take them separately). A typical daily formula for anti-ageing currently looks something like this:

Vitamin A	10,000–20,000 IU
Betacarotene (pro-vitamin A)	100–150 mg
Vitamin C	21–10 grammes
Vitamin B1	200–500 mg
Vitamin B6	200–500 mg
Pantothenic acid	500 mg–1,500 mg

(These B vitamins are always taken together with a tablet supplying the full B complex. Otherwise deficiencies in one or two of the B group might occur over a long period of time.)

Bioflavonoids

	500 mg–1,500 mg of rutin
	500 mg–1,500 mg of hesperidin complex
Vitamin E	400 IU–2,000 IU
Selenomethionine	200 mcg
Zinc picolinate	50 mg

Proteolytic Enzymes – Help for the Future

Behind the first two lines of defence against ageing on a cellular level comes a third which is the most speculative but, in many ways, the most interesting of all. It is that of using substances which reverse the cross-linking process by breaking down the chemical bonds formed through oxidation reactions. This results in the elimination of age-related changes associated with such oxidation – in other words, rejuvenating the body by rectifying the damage already done.

This dream of the age-researcher is very close to becoming a reality. Bjorksten has actually discovered a microbial enzyme – a special strain of the bacillus cerus – which is *proteolytic*, that is, protein-digesting. It can reverse the cross-links formed, for instance, in the tanning process, so that a hide returns to its original soft shape even after having been turned into leather. But the enormous amount of time and money which is needed to bring such a substance on to the market in the form of an anti-ageing drug has so far made this impossible.

Nature's Anti-Ageing Enzymes

There are, however, *proteolytic enzymes* which occur in various foods which some age-experts believe can have a less potent yet still beneficial effect, by dissolving some of the body's cross-linked proteins. To make use of them, they say, all you have to do is eat these foods, on their own and in the raw state. Papain in pawpaw is such an enzyme. It resembles pepsin, the enzyme which breaks down protein in your stomach. It is capable of digesting 35 to 100 times its own weight of protein. Pawpaw has been used medically because of the power of its enzymes: it is applied raw to the skin's surface on sores and surgical incisions which don't seem to heal. The papain breaks down necrotic protein material and allows healing to take place.

The bromelain in raw pineapple is another useful proteolytic enzyme. When you eat either of these fruits raw on an empty stomach and on their own, significant quantities of their proteolytic enzymes enter your bloodstream, according to Dirk Pearson and Sandy Shaw, two age-researchers who advocate their use. This, they say, results in a certain amount of cross-linked and some normal collagen being broken down. Your body will then replace them with new fresh collagen.

There is also some evidence that the anti-oxidant nutrients may to some degree repair damage already done through oxidation reactions. And, although there are as yet no concentrated proteolytic enzymes on the market which have been specifically produced to tackle ageing, these nutrients – through pineapples and pawpaws – are easily available. In addition to making them a regular part of your diet (a couple of pawpaws make an excellent supper instead of the usually heavy meal most people eat in the evenings) you can also apply fresh pawpaw and pineapple direct to the surface of your skin to clear away a lot of old dead cells and leave it looking smooth and sleek. It is in part this principle that lies behind the recent enthusiasm about AHA or fruit acid skin care products.

But, useful though the anti-oxidants may be in helping wage war against ageing on a cellular level, they are certainly no 'cure-all' designed to be used indiscriminately by people who live on junk-food, take tranquillizers and get no exercise. They, like the proteolytic enzymes in certain foods, won't work miracles. No, you need a way of living that encompasses the dimensions of ultra-health, yet is personalized for you alone. Then, added as special bonuses to defeat ageing, they should be *really* effective.

17
The Rejuvenators

IS REJUVENATION POSSIBLE? Can you reverse age-related changes in the body? The average British or American doctor dismisses such questions with a wave of the hand. Yet several hundred of their European counterparts insist they are wrong. A growing number of physicians and age-researchers claim that there are several forms of treatment which used in conjunction with a change in diet and methods for dealing with stress, can help regenerate aged tissues and organs, stimulate a lagging immune system, prolong vitality and restore the equilibrium which modern stress-filled life disrupts. Some of these treatments rely on fresh animal cells injected into the body, others on procaine (a local anaesthetic), still others on DNA or RNA or on glandular extracts taken as you would nutritional supplements. One of the newest and most promising is thymosin – factors taken from the thymus gland. So exciting are the results European practitioners are having with it that many claim it will form the foundation of medicine of the future – an approach to health which, instead of treating specific symptoms, strengthens the body's own defences not only against ageing but against illness. Here are a few of the most well-established of the 'rejuvenators'. Although little formal human research is available to confirm the value of some of the techniques, they are certainly worth looking at.

Anna Aslan's Gerovital-H3
Focus of controversy for more than a generation, Gerovital-H3 is probably the most famous rejuvenation therapy in the world. It was the brain-child of the Romanian physician Anna Aslan, who first

used it to treat the elderly in the early fifties at the Geriatric Institute in Bucharest. Gerovital's use was supported by the Romanian government who provided it for factory workers as a preventative treatment against depression and some of the negative aspects of ageing. It has reportedly been used by many of the world's famous – from John F. Kennedy to W. Somerset Maugham. Aslan claims that the drug has shown itself useful in the treatment of many age-related conditions – from wrinkled skin, greying hair, baldness and sexual dysfunction to arthritis, Parkinson's disease, depression, chronic fatigue, cardiovascular disease and poor memory.

What Is It?

Gerovital-H3 consists of a two per cent solution of procaine hydrochloride, together with traces of potassium metabisulphate, benzoic acid, and disodium phosphate, but its biological activity appears to depend on the procaine – a common drug used extensively in Britain and the United States as a local anaesthetic by dentists and doctors. Procaine is a vasodilator (it expands blood vessels), a thyroid inhibitor and a muscle relaxant, and it has antihistaminic actions. Gerovital-H3 is usually given first by injection and then in a course of tablets as a follow-up treatment. In the body it breaks down into two components which are believed to perform specific functions in the brain and nerve tissues and in other organs: para-aminobenzoic acid (PABA) and diethylami-noethanol (DEAE). PABA, which is a member of the B group of vitamins, stimulates the intestinal flora to produce other vitamins such as thiamine, folic acid and vitamin K. It is often used to protect against sun damage and is a highly effective sunscreen in many suntan products. DEAE is closely related to deanol which has been used as a life extender in animal studies and is one of the components of chlorpromazine, a drug often used to treat old people. It is one of the chemicals involved in the synthesis of choline, which is often praised for its anti-ageing effects on the brain. There are a number of Gerovital-H3 'imitations' around – none as effective, such as the German alternative KH3 – which, in addition to procaine, contains haematoporphyrin, an anti-depressant known to have some toxic effects.

Gerovital as an Anti-Depressant

The drug has continued to arouse controversy for thirty years in Britain and America. This is partly because the protocol of studies done with it in Romania, which show it can extend life and reverse many of the signs of ageing, have not been conducted under what scientists here consider proper controls. There is also considerable hostility in the medical community towards Aslan's treatment simply because, like some of the other rejuvenation therapies, it has been taken by people who have held it to be a 'miracle cure' and of such things physicians are always wary. Many doctors are unwilling to use the treatment, despite the fact that it is very inexpensive, lest they make fools of themselves with their colleagues.

There are a number of animal studies which imply that the drug does indeed prolong life and a few which imply it doesn't. So this aspect of claims made for it remains unsettled. Gerovital-H3 does however seem to be an excellent anti-depressant which, unlike many of the other drugs used to treat depression and anxiety in older people, is relatively (though not absolutely) non-toxic. There have been several controlled studies demonstrating its ability to improve mood in people over fifty. They feel better and more relaxed, and get relief from depression, as well as from some of the pain of chronic inflammation which older people often suffer, such as that in rheumatoid arthritis and degenerative diseases.

How Does It Work?

Used as an anti-depressant, procaine is an anaesthetic and appears to have important actions on the brain's neurotransmitters. It is currently believed to act as an inhibitor of monoaminoxidase (MAO). High levels of MAO occur in many psychiatric disorders, including the kind of depression associated with age. Many of the common anti-depressants are MAO inhibitors (MAOI drugs, as they are known) as well. The significant difference between them and Gerovital-H3 is that they can have serious side-effects such as hypertension, brain haemorrhage, and liver damage. Gerovital-H3 appears to be free from such problems. Instead it modifies the brain's monoamines and makes people feel much better. Its actions on the rest of the body are less well understood.

The Romanian Cure

In eastern Europe every year many people still go to Aslan's centre for a Gerovital-H3 cure. It usually lasts about a fortnight, during which clinical tests are performed, then treatment begun in the form of injections. Patients usually leave with enough of the drug for a year's follow-up self-care. More recently Aslan has used a new product, Asiavital, which is also based on procaine but contains as well 'an activating factor and an anti-arteriosclerosis factor efficient in the prophylaxis and cure of . . . the process of ageing of the central nervous system and the cardiovascular apparatus'. It is usually given together with Gerovital-H3, which is available both in Britain and the United States.

Tackling Genetic Mutations

Many of the rejuvenation therapies such as cell therapy, the Filatov method, organ-specific RNA treatment and the use of organ-specific antisera attempt to do two things. First, they aim to revitalize and rejuvenate the body on a cellular level, thereby reversing the slow-down in cell reproduction and the occurrence of mutations in the DNA (which holds the genetic code) and the RNA (which carries information from the genes for the formation of new protein). Second, they stimulate a lagging immune system. The most famous of all is cell therapy.

Cell Therapy

Live cell therapy used for its anti-ageing properties, like its revolutionary new human counterpart foetal cell surgery, is a simple biological technique which relies on fresh live cells taken from specific embryo tissue – the brain, the liver, the thyroid, and so forth – being injected or 'implanted' into the body of an ailing or ageing person.

What makes such implants valuable is the fact that cells from the unborn are *immunologically naive*. That is, because they are in a primitive state of development, the body does not yet recognize them as its antigens – distinctive proteins which it identifies as foreign and then rejects. That is why, unlike organs transplanted by surgery such as the kidneys or the heart, they cause low or minor immune reactions and therefore no dangerous rejection.

In fact the non-antigenic quality of embryo cells plays an

important role in the development of the life of every mammal. For instance, each of us has a different blood group from our mother and a completely different tissue type and yet, thanks to immunological naivety and to the protection offered by the placenta and its umbilical cord, a child can live at peace in the body of its mother for nine months without either being hurt by her immune reactions or harming her body. So when embryo cells from either animal or human origins are injected into the body, except in very rare cases, it accepts them.

Live cell therapy has ancient antecedents. As far back as 360 BC Aristotle spoke of a group of healing preparations taken from animal or human organs. In the 16th century the Swiss doctor Paracelsus anticipated its basic principles when he said, 'The heart heals the heart, the kidney heals the kidney.' And that is exactly what happens in cell therapy treatment – cells from a foetal liver are used to treat an ailing human liver, for instance, or cells from an unborn spleen are given as treatment for a troubled human spleen. At the beginning of this century a Russian surgeon named Professor Serge Voronoff became famous – even notorious – for implanting cells from apes' testicles in to human males as a treatment for premature ageing and impotence.

Niehans' Magic
The father of modern cell therapy was another controversial doctor – the Swiss surgeon Dr. Paul Niehans. At first Niehans transplanted whole glands from animals into his patients through surgical incisions. Then he found he could simply embed fine slivers of organic tissue into muscle pockets and get the same results. That is, until he discovered a better method: injecting cell suspensions of specific organs, glands and tissues into the buttocks of his patients using large hypodermic needles. His first injection was given in 1931 to a woman suffering from severe convulsions who had been transferred to Niehans' care following an unsuccessful operation on her thyroid gland. Niehans saved her life by giving her a suspension of fresh live cells of animal parathyroid glands. From then on, however, Niehans began to work not only with glands (which were customary in his branch of therapy) but other types of tissues too: heart, liver, brain, etc. Niehans was also the first to use different types of cells from unborn donor animals. For he

recognized, long before any understanding of immune reactions was present in the scientific community, that foetal tissues are more easily tolerated by the patient and also have a more powerful therapeutic effect.

Niehans was an eccentric, outspoken, and opinionated man who fought hard, and some say not always completely honestly, with anyone opposing him. This opposing coupled with the unorthodox (i.e. non-drug) character of the treatment he had developed, gave both the doctor himself and cell therapy a highly controversial image. During his lifetime Niehans' patient records were filled with the names of the rich and famous. He numbered among his clients Churchill, de Gaulle, Eisenhower and Adenauer as well as the Duke and Duchess of Windsor, Picasso, Noël Coward and Somerset Maugham. But what first brought cell therapy to the attention of the world at large was his treatment of Pope Pius XII.

Summoned to the Vatican to inject fresh cells into the critically ailing Pope, Niehans drew popular attention, especially when Pius went to on to live for another four years and insisted that the Swiss doctor had saved his life. Since then live cell therapy has been practised throughout continental Europe and been shown to be successful in the treatment of a wide variety of conditions from Down's Syndrome in children to endocrine disorders and immune-deficiency diseases in adults and (most commonly) as an antidote to premature ageing. In the past fifty years between four million and five million cell therapy treatments have been given in former West Germany alone.

Ways and Means

Although cell therapy is often challenged on the grounds that there is no evidence that it has any beneficial effect on the body, in truth since the early Fifties some 2,000 experiments and clinical reports have been published about it – about half of them from university-based scientists – in European medical publications. These reports not only support the contention that cell therapy can be a highly effective treatment for a wide variety of illnesses and degenerative conditions, but they also indicate that European scientists have considerable understanding of how cell injections function in the body – something which doctors working with the new human-based foetal cell transplants admit they are still at a loss to explain.

Cell therapy consists of several injections made all at once. The injections are made up of cells and tissues from animal embryos which have been carefully chosen to meet the individual needs of the patient. These are determined by the doctor giving the treatment from results of blood and urine tests on the patient and from taking a complete case history. Usually the doctor chooses cells from between 20 and 25 different tissues. They can range from cartilage, connective tissue, lung and bronchi to eye, parathyroid, pituitary, spleen, muscle and thymus – there are nearly forty different possibilities in all. When the patient's 'cocktail' has been prepared from freshly sacrificed animal foetal tissue, it is immediately injected into his or her muscle. The patient is then required to spend at least two or three days in bed so that the biological actions which begin almost immediately can continue without excess stress.

Early on cell therapists believed that cells from each specific tissue migrated to the site of that particular tissue in the human body and settled there. Now researchers know that it is nowhere near as simple as this. Yet what does appear to happen in the living body is, if anything, an even greater miracle. On injection, the embryo tissue particles are loosened and their chromosomes become 'despiralized' within the first 20 minutes. At the same time, human *macrophages* – white blood cells – migrate to the site of the injection to link up with particles from the implanted cells and break them down into smaller particles. The whole process of breakdown takes as little as twenty-four hours, by which time the entire embryo cell material has been degraded and absorbed by these macrophages.

And as this decomposition is taking place, so is something else that's important. The biological materials from the breakdown of embryo cells are being rapidly distributed throughout the body in an exponentially declining curve – the main activity being about forty-eight hours after the first injection.

Radioactive Tracers

Measurements by radioactive tracers indicate that one hour after the injections have been given, a high concentration of the implanted material has reached the various organs of the body, and, even more astonishing, the lion's share of each particular embryo tissue can be found in the specific tissue to which it corresponds in the body. Laboratory investigations even indicate that the degree of absorption of substances from a particular organ or tissue in the body is directly related to the need of that organ for regeneration.

Yet, despite the rapid assimilation of embryo cell material, it can be months before the person receiving cell therapy begins to experience the full benefit of the treatment. This is because cell therapy, unlike drug treatments or the artificial stimulation which comes with using specific hormones, works *biologically*, at the speed of nature. But when improvement does come (in seven out of ten people) it is often dramatic. Over half of patients given the treatment report they feel better within the first two weeks. In fact live cells stimulate repair processes in different organs at different speeds, depending upon how rapidly specific organs or tissues renew themselves. The conditions for which cell therapy has a good reputation include many of the disorders for which foetal-cell transplants are currently being tried: Down's Syndrome, brain damage in early childhood, constitutional sickness and diseases of the immune system such as antibody deficiency syndromes or blood ailments including sickle-cell anaemia. It also appears to work remarkably well in the treatment of skin diseases, neurological disorders including Parkinson's disease, infertility, endocrine imbalances and circulatory problems. But the fields in which clinical reports on cell therapy are most abundant and most glowing are still those of treating age-dependent weaknesses – restoring lost sexual functions, revitalizing the body, banishing arthritis and the rest.

Like foetal-cell transplants, the benefits of cell therapy are based on the ability which immuno-competent embryonic cells, when injected into a living organism, have to stimulate a regeneration of tissues in the recipient body. The mystery is all about how they do this. What do these live cells contain that makes them such potent vehicles for the restoration of normal biological function?

Living Mysteries

Most cell therapists and researchers agree with Professor Franz Schmid, renowned throughout the world for his treatment of children with the technique. He insists that foetal tissue contains a high concentration of biochemical substances, such as enzymes and their substrates, which are designed to bring about the high growth rate of foetal structures.

These substances, when injected into the body, appear to be absorbed by it and made use of in the way it needs to stimulate its own living processes at the most fundamental levels. And when you heighten cell 'aliveness' in such a way, say experts in cell therapy, you ultimately improve the condition of the whole body.

We will probably never know the complete answer to the questions. But one of the factors from embryo tissues which at present appears to be particularly important in bringing about enhancement of energy is the presence of specific growth factors in high concentration in embryo tissue. So when embryo tissue is introduced into the body, these growth factors appear to stimulate the body's repair mechanisms both on a cellular level and in the immune system, resulting in a total revitalization of the organism.

As Dr. Claus Martin, director of the Institute for Live Cell Therapy in Rottach-Egern, Germany, says, 'Live cell therapy is so far our only available form of molecular bio-engineering therapy, so that is why it is probably the best way to stay young and healthier for longer.' In a recent study Martin and his associates compared the complaints and the state of health of more than 370 patients before and six months after treatments. The results indicated that more than 80 per cent of patients valued the therapy as an alleviation of their complaints and an improvement of their state of health.

Filatov's Placental Therapy

At the Filatov Institute in the Ukrainian Black Sea port of Odessa – a city long famed for its rejuvenation therapies – they do a variation on the cell therapy theme: injecting people with human placental tissue suspended in a physiologic saline solution. This is a therapy developed entirely in the former Soviet Union, designed to prevent and treat the symptoms of premature ageing. A very good ten-year research project, examining 130 geriatric patients given the therapy at the institute, showed that they experienced less joint pain, and made fewer complaints about fatigue, weakness and loss of sexual potency, than people who had not received the treatment. A course of treatment consists of three injections of 2 ml of placenta every ten days, then a pause of three to six months before the next three injections. Filatov placental extracts also form the base of some of the best cosmetic products available from continental Europe.

Gland and Tissue Supplements as Rejuvenators

All of these famous 'youth treatments' are based on the use of cells or cell extracts taken from organs or glands and then injected into the body. They are believed to restore a more youthful functioning and appearance to a person. The trouble, however, is that most of them are expensive and some entail time in a clinic (often abroad) under medical supervision. There is, however, another, gentler approach which – although it has been used in biologically-oriented clinics for many years – has only recently become more widely known to the public. It consists of taking 'raw glandulars' – tablets which can be bought without prescription in many healthfood stores. Raw glandulars are tissue-concentrate tablets processed from animal glands and organs. They are taken orally as you might take vitamins or minerals. They are believed to improve the nutritional environment of the body's own glands and organs in much the same way that the more expensive medical treatments do. They are *raw* because they are prepared without heat – usually by freeze-drying – so that any enzymes and beneficial properties of the glands are not destroyed.

Raw glandulars come in two forms – single glandular extracts such as pituitary, thymus, ovary, etc. – and combinations, different ones for men and women, which consist of extracts from several organs or glands in one tablet. Most of the tablets are based on the endocrine glands and each has its own uses. Raw adrenal, for instance, is often used to treat excessive fatigue or nervous exhaustion, low blood pressure, frequent infection, colds and 'flu and other problems associated with excessive prolonged stress; raw pancreas is used for digestive disturbances; and raw thymus specifically to counteract ageing by strengthening the immune system. Organ extracts are available too, such as liver, which is sometimes used in the treatment of arthritis and in blood-sugar disorders, as well as for specific liver problems. The endocrine system, together with the nervous system, carries messages all over the body to regulate metabolism, circulation, growth, repair of tissue, reaction to stress, protection against infection and homeostasis – the constant rebalancing of all bodily functions. It plays a central role in ageing, for when the endocrines are working well, as they tend to in youth, the skin, joints, muscles and organs usually work well too. But when the hormones from one or more of these glands are not in good supply, or when there is a gross imbalance between them, the body is not only more susceptible to illness, but also tends to age more rapidly. The stimulation to endocrine functions from glandular therapy is said to help restore the 'endocrine orchestra' to more efficient youthful functioning and thereby to improve the overall state of the body.

The Controversial Targeting Effect

Primarily made up of protein substances, each glandular supplement puts natural hormones, enzymes, nuclear proteins, vitamins, trace minerals and other active factors into the body. Critics of raw-glandular therapy insist that these reactive substances are denatured in the stomach – broken down by various digestive enzymes so that only the peptides or free amino acids are absorbed into the system. But there is considerable evidence to support the claims of raw-glandular enthusiasts that the tablets are absorbed largely in their original form and that many of their constituent enzymes, hormones, polypeptides, essential fatty acids – and even prostaglandins – do indeed have therapeutic value.

Most of the research and clinical use of raw-glandular therapy has centred in Germany. There scientists such as A. Kment have demonstrated through radioactive-isotope tracing that constituents for glandular tissues can indeed be taken into the body through the digestive system. They are then absorbed by their corresponding gland. The famous (and highly controversial) youth doctor, Ivan Popov, writing in the Journal of the International Academy of Preventative Medicine, claims he used this therapy, '1) in cases of congenital insufficiency; 2) in reduced functional capacity due to disease; and 3) in cases of a decline in functions of organs, groups or function units (regulating circuits) due to ageing.' Like many of the doctors who sing the praises of raw glandulars, Popov insists they need to be combined with other biological approaches, such as vitamin supplement therapy, a good diet and a healthy lifestyle to give best results.

Frank's Nucleic Acid Therapy

Another oral method for rejuvenation has been developed by the New York physician Benjamin Frank, who has used it to treat ageing problems and degenerative diseases. Frank believes that dietary supplements of RNA (usually taken from yeast) together with the vitamins, minerals and other nutritional factors which are metabolically associated with their use in the body, are capable of entering the cells where they increase repair and reverse some symptoms of ageing. He has recently been using RNA in combination with the anti-oxidant nutrients and with the enzyme *superoxide dismutase*, which is known to counteract the destructive effects of oxygen on the cells. In one study, he treated 18 people with 600–2,000 mcg of superoxide dismutase, together with 800–2,000 mg of nucleic acids, 50 mg of B complex vitamins, plus 800 units of vitamin E and 1 gramme of vitamin C. He claims that these patients significantly increased their levels of vitality, and showed improved vision, a diminution of wrinkles on the skin and of grey hair. He insists that his patients eat a diet of foods rich in RNA. Such a diet includes sardines, liver, seafood, mushrooms and wheatgerm. There are numerous animal studies published which support Frank's insistence that RNA from external sources, given orally, is effective in treating ageing and degenerative diseases. RNA has also been shown to be an effective way of improving cognitive functions in animals and there are many clinical reports indicating that it may be capable of improving learning and memory in people – even in cases of senile loss of memory. Some believe that RNA probably has a stimulatory effect on the synthesis or transmission of the neurotransmitter acetylcholine. RNA supplements are also available from some healthfood stores without a prescription. They should not be taken by someone with a tendency to gout and they need to be accompanied by plenty of water, since there is a chance of increasing uric acid levels in the body.

Rejuvenation Now

So there are many possibilities for rejuvenation available now, from mega doses of the anti-oxidant nutrients, to variations of the cell therapy theme to thymosin. There is no reason not to make use of them if and when you feel you need and want to afford them. But none is a panacea. Each one works best when given to a person whose way of living is supportive of high-level health. Indeed some, such as cell therapy, will not even work on people whose bodies are polluted with drugs or alcohol. And, of course, all the rejuvenation therapies should be approached with care and carried out only with professional help. You should remember that, potent as some of these factors can be in their effects on body and mind, none can compare with the power of a nutritionally excellent diet, regular aerobic exercise and a way of managing stress well so that it doesn't manage you. Develop those things and then, if you turn to one of the 'rejuvenators' for help, you may be delighted with the results.

PART SIX

THE ULTRA FACE

18
Skin Fitness Starts Here

YOUR SKIN IS not some delicate covering on the surface of your body which needs constant pampering. It is a dynamically function-ing organ – the largest in your body. How good it looks depends on two things: first, and most important, on the biochemical state of your whole body; second, on how you look after it and protect it from the kind of environmental 'assaults' it is subjected to day after day. Skin accurately reflects your overall state of health. It is also very much affected by how well you deal with stress and all of the other factors important in determining your level of wellness. To have healthy skin which looks great and doesn't age rapidly, you need to get the fundamentals right first. For instance, it is almost impossible to maintain glowing, healthy, attractive skin if you don't exercise regularly. According to a Finnish study published in the *British Journal of Dermatology*, athletes and people who do work out daily tend to have thicker, stronger and more flexible skin. The situation with diet is similar. Living the ultrahealth way is the best possible thing you can do for your skin. That coupled with simple but consistent daily care, plus whatever vitamin or mineral supplements you may need for individual 'problems', will keep it glowing year after year.

Combating Skin Stressors
Your skin is under constant stress. From outside, dry air depletes it of moisture, sunlight ages it, extremes of temperature put strain on its regulatory mechanisms, and air pollutants challenge its integrity. Meanwhile household chemicals – such as ingredients in soaps and bath products, or cosmetics – disrupt its naturally acid pH and

weaken its defences. From the inside it can face equally disruptive influences. For skin is mostly dependent for its health and good looks on the quality of the nutrients supplied to it through the bloodstream and on the proper functioning of enzymes, which in turn are related to your general state of body health and emotions. If your circulatory system is not supplying your skin with the oxygen it needs for efficient cell metabolism, or if certain vitamins or minerals needed for enzyme formation and collagen synthesis are scarce, then your skin suffers. The effects of this kind of deprivation from inside, like those of excessive stress from without, can be measured in real terms – signs of premature ageing, eruptions, excessive dryness or oiliness, and lacklustre skin which no amount of cosmetic treatment can cover up. Looking after your skin so that it can deal with internal and external stressors is a serious but simple business. It demands an awareness of the role nutrients play in skin health and healing, a knowledge of how to clean, protect and treat skin from outside, and a certain amount of respect for what your skin really is – a living, breathing part of your body.

Daily Skin Sense

The skin of men and women differs little, except that men have a beard. Both need the same kind of simple care. In fact, when it comes to keeping skin young-looking, men have the advantage over women for one reason: they shave. At least once a day they gently peel away the outer layers of dried dead cells from their faces while removing the day's growth of beard. Unknowingly they are performing one of the most useful of all techniques for making skin look and feel younger. The simple abrasion of the epidermis can benefit most types of skin, from youthful acne-covered faces to mature lined ones. It is called exfoliation and it makes your skin look clearer and more translucent, which in turn improves the way it refracts light, and softens lines. It can be done with a soap-like cleanser or with a product such as a cream which contains abrasive particles made from sand, polyethylene, silica, bentonite or pumice. But it should be *gentle*. Exfoliation that is too harsh can only damage skin. There are also polyester webs or brushes sold for exfoliating more gently. This can be done using an AHA or fruit acid product. As well as sloughing off dead cells from the skin's surface, exfoliation encourages more rapid cell reproduction beneath, so that your skin looks clearer and fresher and it brings excellent stimulation to the skin – just the kind needed to boost circulation and improve cellular exchange.

The Wash Down

Both men and women can exfoliate while washing or cleansing their face. And cleansing it well is an important part of maintaining fit, healthy skin. This can be done with a mild soap or a detergent cleanser. For a woman who wears makeup, a two-step cleansing process is best, since soap tends not to fully remove the oil-based colours used on her face. Use an oil or cream cleanser first to get rid of every trace of makeup before washing and exfoliating. Men need only the one step: soap.

A word about soaps: there are castile soaps, glycerine soaps, cocoa-butter soaps, deodorant soaps, detergent bars – the list seems endless. The best kind of soap to use is one which doesn't dry your skin. And this has nothing to do with the price you pay for it. Some of the best soaps (or detergent bars, which are just as good) are cheap, and pH-balanced so that they don't disturb your skin's acid mantle. Get the cheapest you can find and stick to it. The best possible way to finish off the cleansing process is with cold water splashed over the surface of the skin. I know men of sixty who have been doing this for 30 years and have skin that looks far younger and firmer than it should at their age. Wearing a mask and snorkel, one well-known actor even plunges his head in a bucket of ice water for five minutes every day. He has superb skin. He is also one of the most fit and firm men you will ever meet.

Keep It Moist

Any kind of wash-off soap or detergent-based cleanser rinses away your skin's natural oils so, unless your skin tends to be excessively oily, you need to use a lubricant afterwards to prevent excessive drying by inhibiting evaporation from the skin's surface and forming a barrier between you and the environment. For men there are a number of good after-shave moisturizers on the market which contain natural moisturizing factors – a chemical cocktail of hydroscopic (moisture-attracting) and hydrating ingredients such as free amino acids, lactates, sugars and electrolytes. These are substances which occur in the skin itself to help it hold water. Similar products are available for women. There is no difference between them except that the male versions are packaged in more 'macho' containers. If your skin tends to be very dry you need more than the standard moisturizing lotion. You should look either for a water-in-oil emulsion which is richer in lipids and longer-lasting in its protective effect than the usual moisturizing lotions, or a triple emulsion moisturizer containing a good supply of essential fatty acids (watch for 'vitamin F' or 'linoleic acid' amongst the ingredients on the label).

The EFA Factor

When applied to the skin these EFAs are drawn into it where they can strengthen cell walls and help restore your skin's ability to retain moisture. Such restoration occurs gradually over a couple of weeks of use. So effective is it that if you stop using these EFAs, your skin's new-found moisture-retention ability remains for quite a while afterwards.

Scientists have discovered that when the body is deficient in EFAs (which happens frequently when people eat a diet high in processed foods), then the cell membranes which are vital for ensuring good retention of moisture become weakened and damaged. Such skin then becomes progressively drier. This kind of fatty acid deficiency is widespread despite the fact that the modern western diet is very high in fats. For so many of the fats we eat have been heated or processed. Chemical or heat processing changes the molecular structure of the lipids from what are known as *cis* fatty acids (which your body can make use of) to *trans* fatty acids. Not only can your body not use trans fatty acids, but they actually block the use of whatever valuable cis fatty acids may be in your diet. The result is that an increasing number of people suffer from dry skin and need a highly effective way to counteract it.

Help for Dry Skin

One of the most effective of all the essential fatty acids for skin is a lipid called gamma linolenic acid (GLA) which occurs in nature in human breast milk and in the oil extracted from the seed of borage or evening primrose. GLA has some remarkable medical properties when taken as a nutritional supplement or rubbed on the skin.

GLA, which our bodies produce from linoleic acid, is an essential element in the making of certain prostaglandins needed for healthy skin and cell growth. The problem is that the body's own

GLA production can be severely impaired by alcohol, a diet that contains too many refined carbohydrates or is too high in animal fat, or simply a difficulty in making the biochemical conversion which some people have. Ready-to-use GLA in the form of a nutritional supplement lets the body get on with making prostaglandins which are important for skin health. Studies show it is an excellent way of combating dry skin, it can produce a significant improvement in eczema and even help eliminate acne.

You can use it two ways – by taking two 500 mg capsules of GLA with each meal (look for one which is encapsulated using nitrogen gas to protect from rancidity) or, after cleansing your face morning and evening, by piercing a capsule and spreading it on instead of a moisturizer. Or do both. It is available from healthfood stores.

How Do Expression Lines and Wrinkles Form?

When a facial muscle contracts habitually again and again, it shortens. But since there is no corresponding shortening of the overlying skin, a line is produced. In effect, what is happening is that the skin is adapting itself to the movement by forming a fold at right angles to the line of muscle contraction. Dermatologists who have studied the histopathology of wrinkles report that there is no difference between the cells in a wrinkle and the cells from the face's smooth areas. Wrinkles are formed entirely because of changes in the collagen 'mattress' beneath the skin's surface. The cross-linking of collagen affects skin in other ways too. When it turns what was a very resilient mattress of connective tissue into a rigid, less well-organized criss-cross of fibres, it tends also to restrict proper cellular exchange in the skin and to reduce the concentration of *glucosaminoglycans* (GAG) – important polymers which appear to serve as a template for the laying down of collagen. So in a kind of vicious circle, one age-related change reinforces another. Some of these collagen changes appear to happen as a natural part of the body's ageing process. Drinking alcohol and smoking cigarettes also brings about the cross-linking of collagen, as does exposure to environmental pollutants. But this cross-linking is most rapidly accelerated by UV light.

Beware of UV Radiation

Researchers can now state with absolute certainty that exposure to

UV light causes your skin to age in exact proportion to the amount of light it has been exposed to. Visible signs of this damage include wrinkling, dryness, mottling, broken blood vessels, thinning and sagging skin. These things don't actually show up on your skin's surface until 10 or 20 years after damage to the underlying tissues has occurred. The exact mechanisms through which this damage takes place are still uncertain, however.

UV radiation falling on your skin appears to be readily absorbed by the nucleic acids in the cells such as the well-known double helix chemical DNA. DNA in the nucleus of every cell is the ingredient which enables it to reproduce itself accurately. UV radiation reaching the DNA can cause errors in the genetic code that result in cell mutations and these errors build up so that skin begins to age prematurely. The risk of skin cancer is also increased. Although there is some possibility of repair by the body's own mechanisms, it is never total.

The Three UV Bands
UV light, which is responsible for making your skin tan, can be divided into three wavebands – UVA, UVB, and UVC depending on the length of the wave and its effect on the body. UVC, the band with the shortest wave, is of no concern for skin because most of the sun's UVC waves are stopped from ever reaching it by the atmosphere which surrounds the earth. Slightly longer than the UVC waves are the UVB. These you hear a lot about because they are the ones mostly responsible for sunburn. They are also the ones which suntan products and *fast* tanning sunbeds either screen out completely or drastically reduce. In advertising copy you will find these UVB rays referred to as 'dangerous' or 'harmful', the implication being that they are the waves you should avoid at all costs. And indeed you should. But the longest of the wavelengths, UVA, is often, very misleadingly, referred to as 'beneficial' or 'helpful' because it does not cause skin to burn.

Stay Away from Artificial Tanning Beds
When you are exposed to UVA alone (the kind you get when you use one of the new sunbeds for artificial tanning), provided the intensity of the light is strong enough, it will rapidly and effectively instigate the tanning process and turn you a golden brown (or whatever

colour you are capable of turning, according to your genes). So far so good. But here's the catch – and it's a big one. UVA light is not the innocent force for good that publicity would have you believe. The world's leading dermatologists warn strongly against repeated exposure to intense UVA light. This is because of all the UV wavebands it penetrates your skin most deeply. And, although for obvious ethical reasons, it is impossible to carry out large-scale research proving the long-term effects of large doses of UVA light on *human* skin, experts are almost unanimous in agreeing that UVA is harmful to the skin. Because of its ability to penetrate deep down into the dermis, it is probably the most important of the three in causing the skin to age. If you value the look of your skin and want to keep it young-looking as the years pass, think twice before undertaking any course in artificial tanning. In ten or fifteen years when the damage you do now would have begun to show, you will be glad you stayed away from it.

Some people believe that a UVA sunbed tan will offer them some protection against sun-related damage later on while they are lying on the beach. This is also untrue. When your body is tanned by UVA alone, two essential steps in the tanning process remain unfinished – the transference of melanin to the keratin layer at the skin's surface and the thickening of the epidermis which produces a protective protein layer. So, despite the false sense of security, a sunbed won't even offer your skin protection against burning in natural light afterwards.

Winning the Battle Against Skin Ageing

If you are to keep your skin looking young and good year after year, effective protection against the effects of ultraviolet light is essential not only while you're lounging on the beach or playing tennis, but all year round every day. Choose a moisturizer which contains both UVA and UVB sunscreens (there are many on the market now) or simply wear a good 'water-resistant' water-in-oil sun lotion on your face instead of a moisturizer. It should have a protective factor of 7 or more. It will last all day and won't wash away just because you get hot and sweaty when you exercise. This is by far the most important thing you can do to keep your skin from ageing quickly. For the ageing process of skin is closely related to the action of light falling on it.

Beware of Skin Hazards

Drinking alcohol can have many ill effects on skin. For instance it vasodilates the tiny blood vessels giving it a red and blotchy look, and it depletes your body's supplies of some of the most important nutritional 'protectors' against ageing skin, including vitamin C and vitamin B1. It also spurs the production of acetaldehyde in the liver which triggers cross-linking.

Caffeine in coffee can bring about similar results while a high-fat diet is a factor in the development of xanthomas, fatty little skin tumours which look unsightly.

External Help for Ageing Skin

Skin care formulations (for both men and women) are becoming increasingly sophisticated and effective. There is also a trend towards ever more specific products to fulfil one purpose at a time – many directly related to combating skin ageing. For instance, a number of companies make products containing active ingredients which increase oxygenation in skin cells or stimulate cell turnover (two functions which slow dramatically as the years pass) so that they more closely resemble that of young skin. Others have begun to address the ageing problem from the point of view of stimulating the rate of repair to the genetic damage that has been done to the cell using anti-oxidant ingredients. They can all be helpful in keeping your skin looking young. But by far the most effective approach to combating skin ageing is an 'internal' one. It depends on the right food, exercise and stress-management lifestyle, coupled perhaps with the use of anti-oxidants and special substances which may help protect the cell's genetic material and the skin's collagen and elastin fibres from cross-linking. Any programme (such as that outlined in Chapter 16) designed for protecting your body from age-related changes will work its wonders on your skin too.

Special Nutrients for Special Purposes

Nutritional supplementation cannot only be useful in helping to retard the signs of ageing skin, it is also useful in treating specific skin problems. For instance, nutritionally aware dermatologists and physicians often recommend for patients with skin problems that in addition to taking a good high-potency nutritional formula of vitamins and minerals (see page 190) they take extra amounts of specific nutrients depending on what skin condition they are trying to overcome. Habitually dry skin, for instance, can benefit by adding evening primrose oil – 1,500 mg to 3,000 mg a day – plus an extra 50–100 mg of vitamin B3 and 25–50 mg of potassium to the standard formula. For acne sufferers an increase in vitamin A or betacarotene, potassium and zinc, are prescribed, and for weak or brittle nails kelp tablets, more B6, C, A, calcium, silicon and magnesium are ordered. This new way of dealing with skin, nail and hair problems can be a powerful force in correcting them.

Interestingly also cosmetic problems with skin, nails and hair can be a useful indication of what kind of nutritional supplementation will benefit the whole body. For instance those white marks beneath some people's fingernails are one of the best indicators that the body is deficient in zinc. Taking supplements of chelated zinc or zinc orotate can not only clear them up, it can also re-establish good overall zinc balance in the body and improve the functioning of many enzymes.

Help for Acne

• **Topical Vitamin A (retinoic acid)** put onto the surface of the skin enters the pores and breaks down oils and bacteria which have accumulated around infected follicles. It also increases the turnover of dead cells on the skin's surface and keeps them from sticking together. But because retinoic acid can redden and irritate the skin it often makes things look worse before skin gets better.

• **Benzoyl Peroxide** is often used together with retinoic acid. It occurs in some of the best over-the-counter preparations for treating acne. The retinoic acid increases the bactericidal qualities of the benzoyl peroxide which also reduces irritation caused by the acid. But it too can be an irritant so it is best to start slowly with small amounts when you begin using it and then increase a bit each day.

• **Flowers of Sulphur and Ice Packs** can be helpful in severe acne. Smooth pieces of ice over the face gently after you have thoroughly washed your skin to reduce inflammation and swelling. Then you can blot skin dry and apply the benzoyl peroxide. Do this twice a day, unless acne is very severe. In that case, mix the benzoyl peroxide with a teaspoon of flowers of sulphur and apply externally.

Gentle Approaches to Troubled Skin

Acne, which affects one in five people at some time in their lives, is a complex problem to treat. It can even be difficult to define. It is usually divided into four categories: first are the simple, mild blackheads which many people get from time to time – some only on certain areas of the face such as the nose and chin where skin tends to be oilier. Second are the larger, more serious blackheads, whiteheads and tiny scattered pimples. More severe is the inflammatory kind of acne which consists of pus-filled pimples from which scarring can result. Finally comes cystic acne which is most damaging and tends to be widespread on the surface of the body. It causes deep and shallow crater-like pits. All kinds of acne respond to the same treatment. The most severe varieties, however, probably need medical care as well as daily external treatment and nutritional support.

Each square inch of your skin contains 95 to 100 oil glands, which in puberty are stimulated to greatly increase their production of sebum by the male hormones, the *androgens*. This is true for both men and women, for although a woman's body produces primarily the female hormones, the *oestrogens*, it also manufactures androgens in the adrenal glands and in special cells of the ovaries. In most women the far greater quantity of oestrogens keeps those androgens well in check. When it doesn't these women, who, like many men, have very high levels of male hormones in their bodies, suffer from pustules, blackheads and cysts.

It is not only the oil which is responsible for eruptions. The overactivity of the skin cells at the basal layer – something also related to these high levels of androgens – also encourages acne. This results in an increased turnover of skin cells and a build-up in skin thickness, while the cells of the skin which line the oil-producing glands and ducts themselves shed excessively. The ducts then become blocked, and the openings which connect the oil-producing glands to the skin's surface get covered over. The trapped oil, together with the skin cell debris and bacteria, then produces ideal conditions for acne to develop.

The Stress Factors

Many factors can aggravate the hormonal imbalances which encourage acne. Samuel Frank, researcher at New York

University, showed for instance that anxiety and anger increase the flow of sebum while periods of tranquillity significantly decrease it. The low levels of oestrogen in a woman's body just before menstruation can have a detrimental effect on skin. Similarly, certain drugs such as salicylates (aspirin), and barbiturates and medications such as lithium and dilantin, can activate acne as can some preparations which contain iodine.

In recent years a number of antibiotics – the tetracyclines and their derivatives – have been used with some success to control acne. They work by reducing the concentration of fatty acids in the skin so that in four to six weeks many people notice considerable improvement. But antibiotics bring problems too. The lengths of dosage involved mean they reduce the level of normal intestinal bacteria which produce important B complex vitamins to nil, leaving the body susceptible to fatigue and stress problems. Sometimes, too, they cause allergy, especially when skin is exposed to sunlight. Finally the beneficial results from such treatment is often not lasting.

Help from Zinc and Vitamin A
Zinc can speed the process of skin healing, encourage collagen synthesis and help clear up blemishes and acne. Low levels of zinc tend to be common amongst acne sufferers. Researchers at Uppsala University Hospital in Sweden found that giving zinc and vitamin A together is successful on its own in clearing up 65 per cent of the cases of acne they treated. Follow-up studies have had similar results. Most doctors treating skin problems in this way use 45–50 mg of zinc in its picolinate form taken three times a day with meals and from 25,000–50,000 IU of vitamin A once a day. Zinc is available from healthfood stores. Eating liver several times a week, or even once a day, is probably the most accessible source of vitamin A. It is doubly useful for people with skin problems because it is so high in the B complex vitamins which are excellent for improving skin health.

Care Now Means Superb Skin Later
Smooth, wrinkle-free skin from one decade to the next is no longer an elusive goal thanks to such knowledge and to the rapidly developing techniques and anti-oxidant supplements available for

holding back the ageing process of skin. But it is what you do *now* for later that matters. Good daily skin care need be neither time-consuming nor expensive. And prevention is a lot easier than trying to repair damage already done. Even that, however, appears to be possible – provided you develop your own individualized ultra-health way of living. The better you feel, the better the biological functioning of your body. And the more successfully you manage stress, the better you'll look.

19
Hair Care:
The Second Revolution

THE LOOK AND condition of hair is something both men and women seem to spend a lot of time worrying about. And rightly so, for hair that's healthy, strong and well cut is an enormous boon to how good you look and how you feel about your image.

The first revolution in hair care – based on new advances in cosmetic chemistry – took place thirty years ago. The second has just begun. Founded on sophisticated new knowledge about how the body's biochemical balance (or imbalance) affects skin and hair, it holds out enormous promise for making healthier and better-looking hair. Warding off or reversing age-related changes to hair, getting rid of dandruff and protecting the body from hair loss are three of the most important areas beginning to bear fruit from the new approach – which works from the inside out. But, let's look at the outside first.

Onwards from the First Revolution
The technological revolution in external hair care products began thirty years ago, when cosmetic scientists discovered that some important changes in the look and feel of hair could be made – provided you found the right ingredients to add to shampoos and conditioners. For instance, they discovered that an alcohol with humectant (water-attracting) properties called glycerol or glycerin, when applied to the hair, would penetrate the cuticle and stabilize a hair's moisture content. It helped each separate strand to draw moisture from the air. This discovery was (and still is) a godsend for dry hair, since it can keep it from becoming brittle and breaking easily. Later scientists found out that the polypeptides obtained

from certain kinds of hydrolysed animal protein, when added to shampoos and conditioners, would soak through the hair shaft and stick to its inside walls. They added strength and body, helped to remove split ends and formed a sheath around lank or thin strands. They could make the whole head of hair look and feel thicker.

Then, cosmetic researchers developed products containing quaternary ammonium compounds. Called 'quats', these compounds have *substantivity* – that is, they can attach themselves to hair fibres and tend to stay there, protecting hair from the ravages of wind, sun and blow-drying far better than the oil-based emulsions which were used in early conditioners. The new non-oily conditioners you can buy are quat-type formulations. They are superb products – particularly for normal and oily hair – with a useful ability to neutralize electrostatic charges in newly shampooed hair. These products will do a lot to improve the condition and look of hair which has been damaged by strong detergents, perming, straightening, tinting or bleaching. All three of these discoveries continue to be important in the wide variety of hair shampoo and treatment products for men and women, and they are available in every price range. Recently not a great deal has happened to increase the cosmetic scientist's knowledge of what can be done to improve hair from the outside. Perhaps in part that is because the main focus of attention in the last few years has been on hair health and how to improve it from within.

Ask Any Horse

Talk to a vet or a horse breeder about the poor condition of your pet's coat and you will get the same answer – change his diet, or give him supplemental vitamins and minerals, or both. These professionals used to dealing with animals know well that the strength, gloss and beauty of an animal's coat depend on how close his diet comes to providing, not just *adequate*, but *optimal* quantities of essential nutrients. When the horse looks poorly, the breeder adds more vitamin B6 or PABA or vitamin A to his feed. In a few weeks' time his coat is thick and gleaming again. It has taken until quite recently for trichologists and doctors to realize that a similar approach to the treatment of human hair can yield the same remarkable improvements. They've started asking, for instance, 'What might be done to stop the kind of changes that happen to hair as the body ages?' And they have begun to formulate nutritional approaches to a lot of other annoying hair problems such as dry brittle hair and dandruff.

Halting Age-Related Changes

As the years pass, certain things tend to happen to hair. The production of sebum decreases so that your hair becomes increasingly dry and brittle. This is particularly a problem in dry climates where, without enough of the natural lubricant produced in the scalp's sebaceous glands, the scales of your hair's outer layer – the cuticle – become raised and flake off. Such flaking makes hair look drab since each strand no longer refracts light the way it did when it had a smooth-lying surface. It also weakens your hair, making it break easily. Another important change which takes place when hair ages is a loss of pigment. The melanin in it decreases, which means your hair loses its intensity of colour and becomes a pale imitation of its former glory. Also, the cuticle becomes more susceptible to damage either chemically, by harsh shampoos, perming lotions or colourants, or mechanically from the heat of a blow-dryer or simply from vigorous brushing. Most of these so-called age-related changes also occur to hair where there is evidence of subclinical mineral or vitamin deficiencies in the body.

Guard Against Mineral Deficiencies

Such deficiencies are becoming increasingly widespread in developed countries because our eating habits are so unbalanced and our convenience foods so depleted of nutritional values. An important area of concern for people who are heavy meat-eaters is that of mineral depletion from excess protein. When a greater portion than 15 to 20 per cent of your daily calories comes from protein-rich foods such as meat, your body can go into what is called a 'negative mineral balance' and you begin to lose important trace elements and minerals from your bones and tissues. At Harvard University in the Department of Nutrition, for example, researchers studied people on a high-protein diet and found that it encouraged osteoporosis – a softening of the bones and a susceptibility to breakage which is particularly common in women after menopause. Many other minerals important to hair strength and good looks, including zinc, magnesium, iron, potassium and selenium, can be leached from your body on a high-protein diet – much to the detriment of your hair. That long-standing notion – still a favourite of books and magazines – that to have beautiful hair you need to eat lots of protein – needs to be abnegated to the status of old wives' tales before yet more damage is done to healthy heads of hair.

Enough protein but *not too much* in your diet is only the beginning of healthy hair. In order to make proper use of your proteins, you have to have sufficient enzymes which break them down into the amino acids your body uses in the formation of hair and other protein-based structures. The formation of many of these enzymes in your body depends on there being enough zinc available. In fact, a low level of zinc is a prime contributor to poor hair, and one of the main reasons why many people, particularly women on the pill and pregnant women, often have hair in poor condition.

The hormonal changes associated with pregnancy, which are mimicked by the contraceptive pill, cause an increase in copper levels in the blood and a decrease in zinc. Copper and zinc are antagonistic. They need to be carefully balanced to maintain a healthy body. Increased oestrogen levels lead to an increased absorption of copper from the intestines and an increased synthesis of copper-binding protein in the liver which results in falling zinc levels. When this occurs, both hair and skin suffer. And because of the overall effects of insufficient zinc on a person's mental and physical health, many doctors now recommend nutritional supplements of zinc and the nutrients to which its use are related – B2, B6, B12, folic acid and vitamin C – for contraceptive pill-takers and mothers-to-be. When these supplements are given either to women or men with hair problems, these conditions often disappear with dramatic speed.

The Magic Foods for Hair
Three foods are of enormous help to hair in protecting it from age-related changes: liver, blackstrap molasses and sea vegetables.

Liver is rich in vitamin A – essential for healthy skin and for the proper functioning of the scalp's sebaceous glands. It also contains a good quantity of many of the B complex vitamins which help guard your hair from premature loss of colour and preserve its sheen and strength, plus many of the essential minerals which are needed to maintain a full shining head of hair.

Take a tablespoon of blackstrap molasses (be sure to buy the unsulphured variety – you can tell if it's unsulphured by the fact that it tastes good – sulphured molasses is revolting) in a bowl of yogurt or porridge or on its own every day. It contains 3.2 milligrams of iron – almost twice what you would get from a cup of raw spinach – and lots of magnesium and calcium. It is also chock-full of many B vitamins including pantothenic acid.

Sea vegetables – seaweed of all varieties – are the single most potent strengthener of hair (and incidentally nails) you can find in nature. They are veritable treasure houses of essential minerals, including organic iodine as well as the B vitamins, and vitamins D, E and K. You can buy many kinds of dried seaweeds to use in vegetable dishes, soups and curries. You can't find a better helper for hair anywhere. Alternatively you can buy kelp tablets to take with each meal. If you opt for the tablets it is important to take enough, since they are not drugs or even concentrated pills, but simply a dried vegetable product. Most people find that 4–6 300 mg tablets with each meal bring enormous benefits to the look and strength of their hair within six to twelve weeks. Like all nutritionally based approaches to good looks, kelp tablets take time to work their wonders. Remember, it may have taken years for a body to become depleted in essential minerals which shows itself in poor hair condition; a few weeks to restore it to a healthy balance is not long to wait.

B Vitamins for Good Colour and Thickness

Men too often suffer from subclinical deficiencies of zinc thanks to an imbalance of zinc and copper in their bodies or the presence of lead in their system. It tends to make them irritable and easily fatigued and stressed. Such a deficiency can be corrected in a few weeks with zinc supplements.

Probably the most important of all the nutrients as far as the health and appearance of your hair are concerned is the B complex range of vitamins. Research has shown that supplements of vitamins such as riboflavin, PABA, biotin, inositol, B6 and pantothenic acid, given to animals whose fur was turning grey, were able to restore the fur to its natural colour. Nutritionist Adelle Davis claimed that supplements of PABA and folic acid are also able to restore the natural colour to greying human hair, while an

American doctor, Benjamin Sieve, has noted that 70 per cent of the people given 200 mg of PABA after each meal show restoration of natural hair colour. Other researchers have found that deficiencies of riboflavin and pantothenic acid can cause naturally curly hair to straighten. Some nutritionists insist that by far the best treatment for dandruff is not dandruff shampoos (which can in the long run make matters worse) but high doses of the B complex range, taken in what we eat.

The best sources of the B vitamins are brewer's yeast, liver, wholegrain cereals and breads and blackstrap molasses. These vitamins – even as supplements – should always be taken in their natural form: that is, extracted from foods, not made chemically in the laboratory. The best way to ensure that you are getting enough is to include plenty of these foods in your regular diet. Eat liver twice a week, eat only wholegrain cereals and breads, stir a teaspoon of brewer's yeast into a glass of fruit juice a couple of times a day. Sugar, alcohol and caffeine destroy the B vitamins and are among the worst things you can consume if you want your hair to stay healthy.

To get the benefit of even one of the B vitamins you need to take it in conjunction with the whole complex. Otherwise, over a period of time, you may develop deficiencies in one or more of the others. The B group of vitamins are water-soluble, so you needn't worry about taking too many of them. Unlike oil-soluble vitamin A, which is stored in the body and an excess of which can cause poisoning, the B group are excreted from the body if taken in greater quantities than you can use. Nutritionists will tell you that the thirteen or more B vitamins are so poorly supplied in the average British or American diet that almost everyone of us lacks some of them. Such complaints as depression, nervousness, fatigue and irritability, in addition to hair troubles, can all point to low levels of this group of nutrients.

Iron, Sulphur and Iodine

Another important nutrient for hair health is iron. If you are anaemic, your hair will tend to be brittle, lustreless and difficult to manage. It will also be thinner than it should be. Women are particularly prone to anaemia and many hair problems are nothing more than an outward manifestation of that condition. If you have been having trouble with your hair and the condition doesn't seem to respond to external treatment from conditioners and protein packs, it is a good idea to have a blood test done by your doctor to eliminate the possibility of anaemia. If you are anaemic, a couple of months on iron therapy will restore your hair.

Two trace elements – sulphur and iodine – are also high on the list of beautiful hair preservers. Sulphur works closely with some of the B vitamins to keep hair strong and glossy. It also has an important relationship with protein. It is part of the amino acids methionine, cystine and cysteine; it is needed for collagen synthesis and is an important constituent of keratin, the tough protein substance from which nails and hair are made. One of the reasons why many men get less than the optimum amount of sulphur in their diet (and why their hair thickness and condition suffers) is because they avoid eating eggs for fear of their cholesterol content. Recent research into the relationship between cholesterol intake and the development of heart disease indicates that our fear of egg-eating has been grossly exaggerated. Cholesterol taken in through foods appears to have far less effect on blood-cholesterol levels than was once believed. Six to eight eggs a week can do wonders for a head of neglected hair, provided the rest of your diet is adequate too.

Iodine is necessary for the healthy functioning of the thyroid gland, and lack of it can have very detrimental effects on your hair. The thyroid governs metabolism in the body and encourages healthy circulation not just in the viscera and muscles but also in the scalp. When circulation there is poor, the hair can weaken and fall out. Oriental women traditionally keep their hair lustrous by adding seaweed (the best nutritional source of iodine you can find) to their dishes. This and their usual diet of fish, soup and salads helps to give them exquisite hair.

The Orthomolecular Approach

The orthomolecular approach is the high-powered branch of the new hair revolution. It is based not only on changing your diet, but on the informed use of specific supplements designed to re-establish biological balance in the cells of the body with specific emphasis on what this can do to improve hair. Nutritionally sophisticated physicians recommend first that anyone interested in improving the state of their hair take a standard multiple vitamin and multiple mineral tablet every day. Such vitamin and mineral formulas, which can be purchased in a healthfood store (buy not the cheapest, but the best you can find), form the foundation of nutritional supplementation on which you can build specific 'treatments'. They are necessary because all vitamins are synergistic – they work together and are interdependent for their health-giving actions on one another. Unless your body has access to all fifty known nutrients necessary for health you cannot expect mega doses of specific nutrients to improve the health and look of your hair – or anything else. Once you have, then you can build specific supplemental groups of nutrients for each problem, from brittle hair in poor condition to prematurely greying hair, dandruff or the prevention of balding. Here are some examples of the kind of regimes that can be designed.

For hair that is dry, brittle and in poor condition. In addition to foundation supplements you might look at:

PABA	150 mg	B1	25 mg
B2	25 mg	B3	50 mg
B5	25 mg	B6	25 mg
B12	50 mg	Folic acid	50 mg
Biotin	300 mcg	Iodine	50 mcg
Evening	6 x		
Primrose	500 mg		
Oil	capsules		

For hair that's greying rapidly or prematurely.

PABA	150 mg	B5	100 mg
B6	25 mg	B2	25 mg
Folic acid	250 mcg	Biotin	400 mcg
Inositol	150 mg	Zinc	25 mg

Nutritional Programme for Hair Improvement
Here is a sample programme for hair improvement; but keep in mind that each person is biochemically an individual and that the quantities given are only a general guideline. Positive results usually show up within a month to six weeks of starting the programme.

- Follow the ultrahealth way of eating which avoids alcohol, caffeine, sugar and drugs, all of which rob your body of B vitamins.

- Take a high-potency B complex vitamin tablet with each meal. Here is a sample formula for guidelines:

B1	175 mg	B2	75 mg
B12	75 mg	Niacinamide	100 mg
Folic acid	400 mg	Pantothenic acid	400 mg
Biotin	150 mcg	Choline	75 mg
PABA	100 mg		

- Eat fresh liver twice a week or stir brewer's yeast (1 tsp to 1 tbsp) into a glass of fresh fruit juice two or three times a day.

- 12–20 mg of zinc picolinate or zinc orotate twice a day with meals.

- Eat 6–8 eggs a week.

- one 300 mg tablets of dried kelp with each meal.

The Dandruff Dilemma

There is more confusion about dandruff than about any other hair problem. Not long ago the American Medical Association studied the incidence of dandruff and found that only 6 per cent of the North American population believe that they have never had dandruff. In fact, Americans spend almost $150 million a year on anti-dandruff shampoos and treatments. A similar situation exists in other western countries. It's the ailment everybody worries about – but nobody knows what the answer is.

Is dandruff really as rampant as we all believe? Not at all. A lot of what is termed 'dandruff' is in fact nothing of the kind. Many dandruff shampoos are unnecessarily used – and, according to some experts in mineral metabolism and heavy metal poisoning, often with consequences that may be very hazardous indeed.

What is Dandruff?

The *stratum corneum* of a normal scalp is made up of 24 to 40 layers of dead dry cells which have moved up from the basal layer of the skin to its surface from which they are sloughed off. The whole process takes about 28 days. This sloughing off of dead cells is a perfectly normal event – they need to flake off in clumps several layers thick. Many people see this flaking appear and assume they have dandruff. Then they begin to use one of the very strong dandruff shampoos to counteract the imagined condition. This only makes matters worse – so much worse that they then feel a need to continue using the product to keep things 'under control', creating a vicious circle. In *real* dandruff, this sloughing process is highly exaggerated so that you are losing flakes from 20 to 50 layers thick. This makes the stratum corneum thinner and exposes fresh young cells to contact with the outside world long before they are hardened and ready for it. It also disrupts the normal pattern of cell turnover – another characteristic of real dandruff.

So far there is no certain proof as to the cause of real dandruff. The prevailing theory is that some kind of microbe or bacterial invasion of the scalp is taking place. But scientific research has not been able to demonstrate yet that this is the case. Despite the uncertainty, clinical tests of the effectiveness of anti-dandruff preparations suggests that anti-bacterial substances in shampoos and treatment products do help a great deal to keep the condition under control. These anti-bacterial ingredients include colloidal sulphur, salicylic acid, resorcinol, cadmium sulphide, zinc sulphide, sodium dioctysulphosuccinate sulphur, and tellurium oxide – you will find one or more listed on the label of commercial shampoos and anti-dandruff creams and lotions. The two considered most effective so far are selenium sulphide and zinc pyrithione.

Cysteine for Hair Protein

Hair is 97 per cent protein, which your body makes out of amino acids, eight of which are essential – they must come from the foods you eat. One of these amino acids – cysteine – is of particular importance to hair. It can be made in the body from another amino acid, methionine. But this conversion takes two vitamins, folic acid and B12, both of which are not always in good supply, particularly among people who have lived on the typical western fare.

Some dermatologists and nutritionists find that giving the single amino acid cysteine in its free form (that is, not part of a long-chain protein molecule) to people who have thin hair or hair in poor condition can make it strong and thicker and more lustrous within a few weeks. Cysteine occurs naturally in good supply in eggs. In supplementary form it should always be taken with vitamin C in a ratio of one part cysteine to at least three times as much vitamin C.

Effective Treatments for Dandruff

Anti-bacterial ingredients such as those I have mentioned are highly toxic. Selenium sulphide, for instance, is very much like arsenic in its actions. Zinc pyrithione and salicylic acid are somewhat less poisonous. It is essential that products containing such ingredients are kept far from the reach of children. So far there are no conclusive studies to show how safe they are for constant use. What is known is that toxic substances can be absorbed through your scalp and there is much concern from nutritionally-sophisticated physicians and experts in heavy metal poisoning that some of the ingredients such as cadmium and selenium used in anti-dandruff products can cause a slow build-up of toxic metals or an imbalance of minerals in the body which may lead to premature ageing and ill health. This is one of the main reasons that many trichologists and physicians have begun to look for other and safer ways to treat both true dandruff and simple flaking scalp. They recommend using a mild shampoo (one marked for frequent or daily use) every day or two, and supplementing your diet with the specific minerals and vitamins known to be helpful to altering for the better the biochemical balance of a body which supports dandruff. In addition to the same basic foundation formula of vitamins and minerals they include: vitamin B6, vitamin B12, selenium – 50 mcg three times a day – and evening primrose oil – two 500 mg capsules three times a day. (They stress that one must not exceed this level of selenium in supplementation as it can be habit-forming and toxic in too high a dose.) Eating liver two or three times a week is also believed to be very helpful for dandruff sufferers.

The Bald Facts

Hair loss is so common that 75 per cent of men over 40 show some signs of baldness. For some men the process begins in their mid-twenties. The causes are many: poor diet or an insufficiency of vitamins, shock, illness, a side-effect of certain drugs or genetically determined 'male-pattern baldness'.

If you are losing your hair, you should find out why before taking any action. It is also important to understand the way hair grows, for not all hair loss is pathological. It is normal to lose a certain amount each day.

How Your Hair Grows

Every hair on your head grows in a three-phase cycle. The *papilla* – the clump of cells at the base of the hair follicle – produces the keratinous cells which are your hair. It is normally well supplied with nutrients and oxygen, thanks to the highly vascular character of the scalp. But if the supply is decreased or interfered with, the hair suffers and hair loss can easily occur. During the first (*anagen*) phase, the hair follicle embeds itself deeply in the vascular scalp to get the nourishment it needs to produce a hair. This phase lasts between two and six years depending on your genetic make-up, your general health and the hormone balance in your body. During this time hair continues to grow from the follicle.

When the anagen phase comes to an end and the hair enters the *catagen* phase, a transitional period occurs which lasts only a few weeks. During this phase, the production of keratin (i.e. the growth of the hair) stops. This means that this particular hair has run its course. It is ready to be shed. Soon it enters the last, or *telogen* phase of the cycle, in which the follicle rests in its contracted state until, after about three months, the hair it contains falls out. This loss causes the follicle to enlarge again and so the cycle continues.

Normal Hair Loss

At any particular time, about 85 per cent of the hairs on your head will be in the anagen phase and the rest in either the telogen or catagen phase. It is normal to lose between 100 and 200 hairs a day. The number of follicles in your scalp never changes. What happens when you lose your hair too rapidly is simply that many of your follicles enter into the telogen phase at once, either as a result of a slowing down of their metabolism or because they shut down altogether. There are many different possible causes of this. A diet high in refined carbohydrates, such as white sugar and white flour, can be a strong contributor to hair damage and loss. Anaemia causes hair loss too, as can low levels of zinc. A lack of any of the B complex vitamins (particularly B1, B2, B6 and B12) can result in lacklustre hair, dandruff, scaling, redness of the scalp and hair loss. Vitamin C is important too, because it maintains the health and strength of the capillaries supplying the follicles. When your levels of vitamin C are too low, this results in perifollicular haemorrhages (the capillaries break and bleed) which means the follicle is deprived of proper nourishment and can die.

Nutritionally-caused hair loss is particularly common among men under high levels of constant stress and those who drink alcohol regularly, since both deplete the body of these nutrients. Smoking, or even spending long periods in smoke-filled atmospheres, also has a detrimental effect on circulation, because of the carbon-monoxide content of cigarette smoke which interferes with the blood's ability to pick up and effectively distribute oxygen to the cells. If you smoke or drink or are under prolonged stress, and you are experiencing excessive hair loss, increase your intake of B complex vitamins and vitamin C considerably.

Hair loss can also be triggered by certain medications – from common aspirin and boric acid (an ingredient in many burn ointments) to steroids (such as cortisone), thyroid medication and anti-coagulants.

Trauma or illness can lead to 'telogen effluvium' – where vast numbers of follicles enter into the telogen phase and are shed all at once. When this happens hair is generally lost in clearly defined patches. New hair growth usually occurs within three months, once the trauma or illness has passed.

Stress and Hair Loss

Alopecia areata, marked by circular bald or thinning spots on the head of women and men, can be the result of acute stress. It is said to be particularly common in women who have trouble expressing anger and who have a tendency to depression. It can be treated internally by a diet high in the anti-stress vitamins, that is, vitamin C and the B complex – and by learning a technique for deep relaxation and practising it regularly. Externally it is treated by rubbing phenol, minoxidil or dinitrechlorobenzene (DTB) on the scalp. Other causes of hair loss include a hyperactive or sluggish thyroid, infection with a high fever, surgery, anaemia, iron deficiency, crash dieting and excessive doses of vitamin A.

Male-Pattern Baldness

One of the most common, and certainly the most worrying kind of hair loss is known as male-pattern baldness. In this condition, the hair does not fall out all at once, but gradually becomes thin and stunted and then disappears. MPB usually occurs in a regular pattern – with the greatest loss in the front and centre of the scalp forming a kind of horseshoe of hair at the sides and back. In spite of the hundreds of formulas (herbal and otherwise) which exist, in cases of MPB there is no sure way to encourage new hair growth by applying tonics from the outside. However, the act of applying a tonic *can* help, simply because it involves massaging the scalp deeply, which improves circulation to the follicles and stimulates their metabolism. But you can do it just as well without the tonic. Here's how:

Press your fingertips and the part of your hand just below your thumb into your scalp at the sides and, keeping them in the same place, rotate them in small circles. You will be moving your scalp, not your fingers – it is important that your fingers stay in the same place to stimulate circulation and so that you are not pulling at your hair. After you have worked in one position on the scalp for about 30 seconds, remove your hands and take up a new position rotating your fingertips firmly for another 30 seconds until you have covered the whole scalp. The whole treatment will not take more than three minutes. Neck tension can also contribute to poor scalp circulation. Here an electric vibrator used on your neck, shoulders and head can be a good investment.

Curiously, a massage cream which has proved helpful in stimulating regrowth is a cream containing the male hormone testosterone – the very hormone which systematically triggers MPB in the first place. American dermatologist Dr. A. M. Klingman used the technique on the heads of 21 balding men between the ages of 29 and 78. He applied the cream to the scalp once a day over a five-month period. In sixteen cases regrowth appeared, but only in the areas of the scalp where the cream had been applied. It appears that testosterone applied locally somehow rejuvenates the hair follicles, encouraging them to take up normal functioning once again.

The Case for Transplants

A transplant is a surgical technique which involves skin grafting. It is done with a punch which takes plugs from areas of the scalp rich in hair, each about 3½ mm in diameter, and containing eight to ten follicles. The plugs are removed from the scalp, cleared of any excess fat and put into holes which have been made with the same punch in thinning or bald areas. Each transplant is spaced at least 3½ mm from its neighbours in order not to disrupt the blood supply and impede healing. Soon after they are put in, the shock of transplanting pushes the follicles into the telogen stage of the growth cycle and the hairs fall out. But within about three months, new anagen hairs begin to grow from them, and the scalp begins to look normal.

Transplanting is usually done under a local anaesthetic. The technique is expensive and results are slow to show themselves. You need about a hundred grafts to replant a receding hair line, two to four hundred if you are really balding. The surgeon or dermatologist usually does about twenty to fifty grafts at a time in sessions from a couple of weeks to three months apart. One disadvantage of the technique is that it gives a rather tufted appearance – which is almost inevitable because of the spaces necessarily left between each graft. Another problem is that successive 'families' of grafts, put in to fill up the gaps between those already there, have less chance of surviving and producing hairs because of the formation of scar tissue in the scalp from the first family.

Alternatives

Because of these disadvantages, several alternatives to transplants have been tried in recent years, the most successful of which so far is the flap rotation technique. With transplants, at most three to five hundred grafts are done, with a yield of somewhere between five and seven-and-a-half thousand surviving hairs. The number of follicles moved and the number of surviving hairs is far greater with the flap rotation technique. Flaps are taken from the sides of the head and moved towards the front hairline to reproduce the look of the original hairline. Each flap is 3½ to 4cm wide and can be as long as 25 cm. It will contain an average of eight to ten thousand hairs. Usually two flaps are all that are necessary – which means a total survival of up to twenty thousand hairs. Flap rotation is also done under local anaesthetic, usually in two sessions with a week between them. The hair does not have to be cut, nor do you get the immediate hair loss which you get with transplants. So after ten days, you have a pretty good-looking new area of hair. Since the vascular supply to the area from which the flaps are taken, near the neck, is particularly rich, the new hair often flourishes. And this area can be stitched in such a way that you don't get a bald patch left. Flap rotation needs to be done by the very best plastic surgeon you can find.

Another alternative is hair weaving. Your own hair is interwoven with teflon threads to create a mesh-like base at the scalp where the hair is thin and hanks of matching hair are attached to the base. Since this is not a surgical technique, it has the advantage of immediate results – your hair looks thicker right away. And you can sleep, swim and shower without being afraid it will fall out. However, hair weaving has some definite disadvantages too. The weave has to be reknotted close to the scalp every few weeks. If you suffer from dandruff it often makes the condition worse. It occasionally also causes *traction alopecia*, baldness which is the result of constant pulling on the hairs.

There are some new nutritional approaches to MPB as well. They, like the other treatments outlined for hair problems, are based on a foundation multi-supplement formula of all the important vitamins and minerals, plus extra quantities of nutrients known to be specifically involved in hair growth and the health of the follicles:

Choline	1,000 mg	Inositol	1,000 mg
B5	200 mg	B6	25 mg
Folic acid	500 mg	PABA	200 mg
Biotin	500 mg	Vitamin C	1,000 mg

Anti-Oxidants to the Rescue

But in many ways the most interesting of the new ways of dealing with MPB is that of using specific anti-oxidant nutrients – an approach which looks at the problem as a symptom of ageing and aims to retard that process. American age-researcher Dirk Pearson uses, in addition to the nutrients specific to preventing hair loss, massive doses of anti-oxidants – from vitamin A, C, and E to those used for retarding spoilage in foods: BHT, plus specific free amino acids such as L-cysteine. This, he claims, has had a remarkable effect on his (and others') male-pattern baldness. He had more hair in his late thirties than in his mid-twenties. And although his methods are extreme in the eyes of more conservative scientists, such experiments tend to pave the way for the more moderate and sensible use of similar substances in the future. They, if you like, are the avant-garde of the second revolution in hair care – an exciting internal approach to hair care and the correction of hair problems which gains momentum every year. There is no reason your hair shouldn't look healthy and thick well into your seventies.

20
The Professional Touch

JUST AS MANY good anti-ageing treatments are available for mind and body, so there are a number of useful professional techniques for making your face look great as the years pass or for correcting problems. They range from 'conventional' plastic surgery to the use of collagen and silicon implants, lasers and electro-acupuncture. Each has its uses. Some also have serious drawbacks. These techniques are not 'cure-alls'. Even the best cosmetic surgery can look frightful after a few months if your skin is in poor condition and your diet does not give you a high level of nutritional support. They are like the icing on the cake to finish off an ultrahealth way of life and banish little imperfections. Let's look at face lifts first.

Does Your Face Need a Lift?
Probably not. Certainly not until you have completely exhausted all other possibilities for improving the texture and tone of your skin. Once the province of wealthy or neurotic women, face lifts are rapidly becoming middle-class, middle-age status symbols for men and women alike. Once you have the two cars, the suburban house and the successful image (so the thinking goes) cosmetic surgery is next on the list. But face lifts are decidedly *not* what your dreams are made of. They are costly, risky and painful. They require not only the mechanical skills of the surgeon but the aesthetic ones of a sculptor if you are really going to look superb afterwards. And there are not that many medical Michelangelos about these days. Yet, properly done, just the right operation done in just the right way can bring enormous positive benefits to an ageing face. Cosmetic surgery may not make you look more beautiful but it can make you

look a lot healthier and younger provided you go into it with your eyes open. To be a good candidate for face surgery you need to have realistic expectations of results, not be overweight and not be looking towards cosmetic surgery to satisfy needs which are not really related to it – such as the need for self-esteem or for a new sexual partner. A revitalized face does not automatically result in a revitalized lifestyle.

Here are a few of the newer and more interesting procedures and what they are good for:

The Classic Face Lift and Its Newer Variations. The classic face lift involves the tightening of the skin and the lifting of the facia beneath. It is usually done under general anaesthetic and takes from two to four hours to complete. The operation entails incisions made at the temple extending down in front of the ear, hugging the earlobe and going across the mastoid bone into the hair. From the incisions the facia and skin are drawn up to remove the slack, the tension carefully adjusted and excess skin cut away. After being carefully moulded to the face, your skin is secured with tiny stitches around the hairline and ears to hold it in place. You usually spend 48 hours in hospital and end up with a face which is swollen and livid for a fortnight.

Newer, more sophisticated, techniques for face lifting such as SMAS (which stands for Superficial Musculo-Aponeurotic System) have evolved that give a more individualized look. For instance, the surgeon may not only work on the skin but on the underlying musculature in the jaw and neck area to give a firmer, smoother line when it's finished. He can extend his hairline incision and do a radical neck lift if necessary to eliminate a crepy throat. He can take away extra skin and fat to create a better chin line or even add an implant to the chin area or use cheek implants. This gives longer-lasting results but needs to be done by a master surgeon so the likelihood of damaging the important vagus nerve in the process is minimized.

Some surgeons like to do a chemical peel or dermabrasion after a face lift to remove fine lines around the mouth and smooth out irregular pigmentation.

The Partial Lifts. There are two types: *segmental meloplasty* for the jaw and neckline and the 'mini' face lift which is simply a 'temple tuck' that removes a piece of skin from the temple area. The first procedure works well for people whose main problem lies in a sagging jaw and neck area. It is usually done in the surgeon's office instead of a hospital and recovery is quicker than from a full face lift. The second – the 'mini lift' is something to stay away from. It usually only lasts a few months and can leave you with a broad scar.

Help for Eyes. Used to correct fullness or bags around the eyes, *blepharoplasty* involves the removal of excess fatty tissue and skin from hairline incisions usually made in the natural folds of the skin so you can't see them. Dermabrasion or chemical peels are often used to improve the look of fine wrinkles in the eye area as well.

There are many variations on the eye lift theme. For instance the surgeon can remove a strip of muscle to make a natural-looking fold above the eye, enlarge the contour of the eye orbit by taking away some of the bone or lift droopy eyes to give them a happier expression. Many surgeons now flatten the muscle which surrounds the eye to help eliminate crows' feet more effectively than could be done before.

The Nose Job. Happily the idea that everyone looks great with a small (and, in the case of a woman, turned-up as well) nose is passing. Nowadays surgeons go for noses that are larger and fit better with the face they are put on. *Rhinoplasty* is a delicate operation. It is probably the most difficult cosmetic surgery procedure in terms of estimating what the final results will look like. In the case of other procedures the surgeon can at least see what he is doing. With nose surgery he is working much more by touch. If he happens to inadvertently tear a nerve high up in the nose it can result in damage that is permanent and untreatable. It also has one of the longest recovery periods in plastic surgery. I would think hard before deciding to embark on nose surgery and if you do, be sure you have the very best plastic surgeon you can find and that you are very sure what you want.

The Brow Lift. To tighten skin over the eyebrows (which the classic face lift can do little for) surgeons have developed a way of making incisions above them and then lifting the brow so it gives a face a younger look. But this does produce scars (no matter how tiny) which are visible. Alternatively, the surgeon can use an incision behind the hairline to flatten the deep creases in the brow and smooth out frown lines as well as raise the eyebrow slightly. But all of this can result in a rather expressionless face.

How Do You Find a Good Surgeon?

Ideally by word of mouth. Knowing people who have had cosmetic surgery and been pleased with the results is best. The advertisements for clinics where they do cosmetic surgery are a poor bet. You have no idea what kind of surgeon they channel their inquiries through. Neither are the numerous bogus societies or plastic surgery 'advisory services' of much use: looked at closely, they tend to be self-serving set-ups for second-rate surgeons. Your family doctor can be helpful if he is sympathetic to your wish for surgery. If not, keep asking people until you find someone you like the look of who likes what his or her surgeon was able to do. When you go to see a prospective surgeon ask lots of questions. Anyone who is unwilling to deal personally in depth with your inquiries is someone you don't want operating on you anyway. Ask the surgeon about his (or her) credentials, how many of the different kinds of procedures he carries out in a week, and exactly what you are to expect if he operates on you. Some surgeons are particularly good with some procedures. Find out his specialities. Look at before and after photographs of people he has worked on. Then listen to your instincts about him before giving the go-ahead.

What are the Dangers?

There are many but in the hands of a master surgeon complications tend to occur only infrequently. A haematoma is one. It occurs when blood collects under the skin, looking at first like a huge black and blue mark. It happens to about 8 per cent of face lift patients. Avoiding all alcohol and drugs – even aspirin – for a fortnight before surgery will help you avoid it. Nerve injuries are rare but they can occur in the forehead or cheek, making the face flaccid and without expression on one side. And of course there are always the dangers implicit in any operation where general anaesthesia is used: the patient can vomit and risk congesting the lungs, or fluctuating blood pressure can result in sustained bleeding. Postoperative problems can also occur if the skin is stretched too tight.

The notion of eyes that don't close after cosmetic surgery or a mouth that is in a constant smile because it won't relax is not just a fantasy dreamed up by humorous cartoonists. This does happen. Choose your surgeon carefully to make sure it doesn't happen to you. Finally, many people suffer from depression after surgery – partly because of the long-term after-effects of the anaesthetics and pain killers they take, partly because their final results don't come up to their dream of 'youth-restored-by-the-scalpel'. If you approach the whole question of plastic surgery unemotionally and realistically, you should not be one of them.

The Aesthetic Syringe

Despite all the new advances in plastic surgery, such problems as acne, surgical scars, deep frown lines, deep smile lines and other fine depressions have been difficult to treat adequately. Implanting a highly purified form of soluble collagen just beneath the skin promises to change all that. Known as *collagen implants*, the new system came originally from research done at Stanford University, where scientists developed a new way of processing bovine collagen into an odourless, whitish substance with the consistency of soft paste. The collagen is suspended in a saline solution and mixed with lidocaine – a local anaesthetic. It is injected with very fine syringes into wrinkles and scars on the face – with remarkably good results. For instance, a plastic surgeon can obliterate a frown line by placing his needle into the dermis at one end of a furrow and sliding it carefully under the skin to the end of the depression, then slowly drawing it back again, all the while injecting the implant which fills the depression as he goes. Then he repeats the same procedure on the same line only more superficially. This fills the depression and raises the skin to the level of the surrounding tissue. The procedure causes only minor redness which disappears in a few days. It can be carried out in a few minutes in a dermatologist's or plastic surgeon's office. Then gradually over the next few weeks the injected collagen becomes incorporated into the body as its own tissue. Silicon is another substance which can be injected into fine lines to smooth them out. Its use is illegal in the United States, but it is still used in Europe. In the hands of a skilled surgeon, such as Dev Basra in

London, silicon is virtually permanent in its effects. 'I prefer it for fine lines around the mouth,' says Basra. 'Collagen just doesn't last. Unlike silicon you have to re-inject it every 2 or 3 months. As far as the dangers of "migration" of the silicon are concerned, they are very slight, for you are using such small quantities.'

Banish Fine Lines
This new treatment is useful for filling in a scar or smoothing out fine lines – like those which appear around the mouth which are hard to treat with plastic surgery. But collagen implants are no substitute for plastic surgery. They will not remove slack skin nor will they tighten sagging contours. They are, however, very good for what plastic surgery has trouble treating. These collagen implants have been carefully formulated to minimize allergic reactions (research shows they occur in only 1.3 per cent of cases), but the treatment must be carried out by a doctor or surgeon with considerable dexterity and the patient must be allergically tested a week or two before. This is done by having an injection of the collagen in the arm and then carefully checking for any signs of allergy. If there are any then you must not have the injections. The treatment is also expensive.

Face Peels
Even the Egyptians knew about face peels. They used salt, alabaster, pumice and animal fats to smooth the surface of male and female skins and make them more attractive. The modern high-technology version of skin peels involves the use of chemicals such as salicylic acid, resorcin, and – best known – phenol and trichloroacetic acid (TCA).

They are designed to eliminate fine lines on the face and they work best on fair-complexioned, thin-skinned people with fine wrinkles. These chemicals are mixed with other substances such as Croton oil, liquefied soap and distilled water and then spread on the face where they cause deliberate damage to the skin. They create a controlled wound akin to a second-degree burn. First your skin turns white, then red. Then, at just the right moment, the burning chemicals are neutralized. A crust gradually forms from underlying tissue and after two or three days new cells start to form. After 10 days to two weeks the skin heals, leaving it smoother and fuller and making lines less conspicuous. The peeling itself takes from half an hour to an hour and is usually done in the surgeon's office. It can be painful for several days. The new skin which emerges after a peel shows less pigmentation, and fewer signs of age, freckles and wrinkles. It also tends to be thinner and needs to be carefully protected from the sun, and in women, from other factors which cause pigmentation – such as oral contraceptives and pregnancy – for the next six months.

When chemical peels were first done, the results were inconsistent. Now, thanks to experience and better substances used, they tend to be much better (although they should never, of course, be undertaken without careful thought and professional help). TCA can be used to give only a light peel, taking off the outermost part of the epidermis. This is particularly helpful for removing uneven pigmentation when it is used in very light concentration (15–20 per cent), but it does little to alter the look of long-term wrinkles. A heavier TCA peel is very much like a phenol one. It involves a short procedure with intense stinging for a few minutes and then the slow period of healing afterwards. Some surgeons like to do a series of light TCA peels. The prices of peels vary considerably from doctor to doctor but they are relatively inexpensive compared with face lifts. And while they are no replacement for the tightening and smoothing action which a face lift has on contours and sagging muscles, they can remove fine lines and they can improve the look of skin with mild acne scars on it. The results of a chemical peel usually last about five years. Chemical peels are of no use in treating large pores and are not recommended for broken blood vessels. Your skin will be slightly lighter in colour after a peel. I am personally very wary of peels since I have seen too many that have gone wrong.

Dermabrasion

In many ways similar to a peel, dermabrasion can go beyond it in that it affects not only fine wrinkles but deeper acne scars and sun spots (*lentigines*). You can have it on almost any part of the body, not only on the face. Dermabrasion can be used to treat frown lines, smile lines, vertical wrinkles, naso-labial lines and fine lines around the mouth. It is done with a dermabrader or planer – which looks like a dentist's drill, complete with different brushes, serrated wheels, fraises and cylinders, all for removing the surface layers of the skin. It is done on skin that has first been painted with a purple dye to show the surgeon where the deeper recesses he is treating are. It is then sprayed with freon, an anaesthetic that temporarily freezes the skin surface. Patients who have had the treatment claim it is not very painful. However, there is a burning sensation, which a cream containing a local anaesthetic such as lidocaine alleviates. The oozing of plasma can go on for a couple of days afterwards and then crusts are formed which loosen in a week or ten days and fall off. They reveal new pink, swollen skin beneath.

Dermabrasion is often used after a chemical peel on areas of the face that need further treatment. The results from this treatment are now much better than they were in the Fifties when it first came in; however there is always the possibility of scarring if the surgeon planes too deeply. Occasionally uneven pigmentation results, and infection is possible (but seldom occurs). After both a peel and dermabrasion you can get a spate of white cyst-like pinpoints called *milia* on the skin which eventually go away by themselves. The doctor can, however, open them with a fine needle and drain them – a painless and quick procedure. You need to figure on ten days to two weeks after a peel or dermabrasion before you are ready to enter the land of the living again. Then a little makeup (even for men) can hide any remaining redness until it leaves.

Laser Therapy
'Port wine' stains, strawberry birth marks and other disfiguring blemishes caused by abnormal concentrations of capillaries beneath the skin surface used to be a matter for concealment alone. Now the argon laser – a finely focused hot beam of light able to burn tissue at incredible speed and with exceptional precision – can treat many of these disfigurations easily, painlessly and in the doctor's office. An argon laser of the proper amplitude can completely wipe out about 15 per cent of these discolourations and dramatically bleach out another 70 per cent. The laser has to be used by skilled hands, however, since it can do damage if not handled wisely.

There are also other kinds of lasers – called cold beam lasers. One, the helium-neon laser, is used cosmetically to improve the look of ageing skin. It is not as dangerous as hot lasers and tends to be used on specific points on the face, many of which correspond to acupuncture points. This 'non-surgical lift' consists of beaming these points with the laser light then directing it along facial lines on the forehead, around the eyes, cheeks and mouth. Finally the entire face is gently bathed in the light. The whole procedure takes between twenty minutes and half an hour. You can usually see a face change colour as circulation improves. Some kinds of laser are also used on the body to treat stretch marks and other minor disfigurations such as scars. These laser sessions are said to improve muscle tone, increase circulation and smooth out fine lines. So far no one has been able to explain exactly why.

Some people seem to get very good results after a series of cold beam treatments (which are usually given in series of ten with a 'booster' every three to six months). They claim to look much younger afterwards. Others have been sorely disappointed. Certainly this kind of laser therapy does not do well on someone who drinks heavily, smokes or is on long-term drug therapy. Its use for cosmetic purposes is still in the developmental stages. It will probably be a few years before it is possible to establish just what kind of laser works best for what.

The Acupuncture Lift

Akin to the cold beam laser treatment is an excellent form of acupuncture face therapy given to tone muscles, improve skin colour, and increase smoothness. It consists of using 10 to 12 needles inserted at specific sites on the face (and occasionally the body as well) just below the skin's surface. The needles are hair fine and cause no real pain – indeed many people find the whole procedure highly pleasant and relaxing, probably because of the effect that acupuncture needles can have on encouraging the production of endorphins in the brain which make you feel 'calm but high'. Your face is almost immediately suffused with pleasant warmth and relaxation which often continues for hours afterwards. The sites for the needles vary from person to person since they are chosen to rebalance the bodily energies along the acupuncture meridians as well as for the local effects they have on the face. The procedure usually lasts about half an hour and has to be repeated five or six times at weekly intervals in order for results (in terms of better tone, firmer muscles, better circulation and general improvement in the look of skin) to last. Then you need a touch-up treatment or two every three to six months, depending on what kind of general health you are in and how old your skin is. It is important not to drink any alcohol or take any drugs before a treatment since they can throw the energy in the body with which the acupuncturist is working very much out of balance. The more overall natural resilience you have – the closer you approach an ultrahealth way of living – the better are the results from the acupuncture lift and the longer they last.

When needles are removed your face is usually given a gentle massage using a mixture of natural oils and herbs or aloe vera to moisturize the skin. In addition to their firming actions on the muscles, the needles seem to dilate blood vessels and step up circulation, which may also increase moisture levels in the epidermis and soften fine lines. Some practitioners use electro-acupuncture – a transcutaneous stimulator powered by a nine-volt battery – instead of needles. This is not a treatment which should be given by an unskilled practitioner because the points need to be carefully chosen, keeping the overall energetic condition of your body in mind, and this takes considerable skill. The acupuncture lift is, however, a superb natural treatment which, unlike some of the other professional alternatives for improving good looks, is very much in keeping with the ultrahealth concept of treating the total person. It can leave you feeling as good as you look.

PART SEVEN

THE BODY BEAUTIFUL

21
Body Freedom

HOW DO YOU feel about your body? Is it a source of pleasure and pride to you? A burden to be borne? A matter of indifference? A 'good runner' which always seems to do what you ask of it? Or is it something on which you are not sure you can depend? Most people feel differently at different times, but for some reason we westerners tend to have slightly uneasy feelings. Perhaps because of the cultural models we inherited from the Greeks which separate 'body' – the physical presence – from 'soul' – the 'real' person, we tend to have a somewhat schizoid attitude towards the body. We tend either to treat it as an object and then alternate between narcissistically indulging and continually neglecting it, or we seem to dissociate from it altogether.

Your body is important. It is the medium through which you experience reality. Your sense of aliveness and vitality, peace and relaxation, joy, sexuality, power and even intellectual enjoyment are all experienced through your physical body. The more alive it is, the more intense your sensation, the more rich your experience of life. Treatments which you can carry out on the surface of your body with such things as water, oils, clays or skin brushing can profoundly influence your state of wellbeing – mentally and physically. They can improve lymphatic drainage by clearing away wastes that have been stored in the system, pep you up when you're tired and relax you when you're stressed. An ultrahealthy body is a finely-tuned instrument. It is sensitive but strong – a body which feels comfortably in tune with the earth on which it stands, yet free to move, to dance, to feel, to experience joy and pain fully. How does it become that way?

ldeally it should always have been. The child born naturally, without trauma or drugs, who enters a safe and welcoming world and has a good bond with its mother, probably already has such a body. It moves fluidly, it experiences emotion and sensation richly and it is fully expressive – both in its shape and its movements – of the nature of its personality. The trouble is that in most of us our natural aliveness and bodily freedom become distorted or truncated by traumas which tighten muscles and damp down sensory input. Some people find themselves oppressed by living in a world which is not really life-nurturing. This is a not uncommon feeling of younger adults. All of these things are felt through the body and can leave their 'scars' on your physical way of being. Then, instead of maintaining the sensitivity and responsiveness which was its birthright, your body slowly becomes 'deadened'. It is a deadness which expresses itself in many ways – from rigidity or strange postural attitudes and gaits to flaccidity – muscles which appear lifeless and skin which is lacklustre.

Reclaiming and Nurturing Your Body

One of the most remarkable things about the human body is its plasticity. Unlike a machine, to which it is often likened, a body can change its shape and ways of movement, it can collect poisons in the tissues where they decrease vitality and promote illness or it can be encouraged to give up these poisons and become more alive, strong and beautiful. You can take a twisted, strained body or one without a great capacity for feeling physical pleasure and gradually over a period of months, reclaim its 'aliveness' and its natural good looks.

There are many useful techniques for doing this. Regular aerobic exercise is one. So is the Alexander Technique. Yoga too can be useful – if it is practised well. There are also many professional disciplines which can help such as the bioenergetic therapies, touch for health and Rolfing or structural integration. But there are also a number of things which you can do for yourself day to day to reawaken body vitality, improve the look and feel of skin and even alter the way you use your body as well as the way you feel about it – and they are enormously worthwhile. For, when your body feels more alive, more responsive and stronger, so do you.

The healing of this culturally inherited mind-body split is a slow, but totally necessary, process in order to achieve the kind of integration which makes high-level wellness possible. Many of the techniques useful for bringing it about – such as the clay and seaplant treatments, massage, water therapy, breathing exercises – can be a lot of fun and can leave you feeling great when you use them, quite apart from the long-lasting benefits they promise. Also, taking time occasionally for them can be an excellent method of de-stressing, allowing you to get away from any leaning towards becoming an 'automaton' – a tendency we all have to some degree – and to take a look at who you are and where you are going. This too is an important part of the ultrahealth way of life.

Water Works Superbly

For instance a simple thing like water which you come in contact with every day can be used for its transformative and vitality increasing properties. It takes almost no time at all. Applications of hot and cold water have become standard therapy for aches and pains for revitalizing the body in continental Europe, thanks to the pioneering work of Father Sebastian Kneipp, the Bavarian parish priest who strengthened his own less-than-hearty health with the healing powers of water and then went on to develop a whole system of treatment, using it to dissolve toxic wastes in the body and to strengthen the entire system. Many of Kneipp's techniques are excellent for bringing vitality and a sense of aliveness. He claimed that the easiest ways of 'hardening and bracing the system' were to walk barefoot: on wet grass or stones: on freshly fallen snow: in cold water up to your knees. Such a notion may sound strange to someone who has never tried it but it can be enormously invigorating – even on winter mornings. I know doctors who use it to increase a patient's resistance to illness, with excellent results. The secret is to spend only a few minutes (from 3–5) walking barefoot in this way, to make sure that you keep shoes and socks dry, and that you replace them immediately afterwards. If they too are allowed to get damp you miss out on the stimulating effect of the contact with the cold dampness and can deplete your body of energy instead of revitalizing or strengthening it. This is the secret of using cold water applications on the body. You need to be warm to begin with and you must keep warm and dry afterwards. Contact with cold water in these circumstances first causes constriction of the blood vessels, momentarily driving the blood inwards. Then, the moment it is stopped, the blood rushes to the surface of the skin, warming it.

A Daily Bid for Vitality

The same principles apply to any kind of cold shower or cold sitz bath. One of the best possible ways of waking up each morning and getting yourself going for the day ahead is to brush your dry skin down well with a dry hemp glove (a loofah is just not strong enough for this) or a natural vegetable bristle bath brush and then to step into a warm shower. As soon as the warmth of the water has suffused your body and you are really comfortable, switch from 'warm' to 'cold' and remain there for only half a minute (no more) making sure that your body all over gets covered with the cold spray. Emerge from the shower, dry yourself briskly and dress warmly. It is important that the bathroom is warm and that you begin very slowly with only, say, 10 seconds of cold water at first, gradually increasing it to half a minute as you become used to it. (You will be surprised at how quickly this can happen.) It will make your body feel alive and tingling, increase your stamina and, according to the European doctors who often recommend it, it can even heighten your resistance to colds and 'flu.

The Cold Sitz Bath for Perfect Sleep

A variation on the cold water theme, the cold sitz bath is one of the best ways of relaxing quickly and making yourself ready for sleep. It is another technique, the effectiveness of which you probably won't believe until you have tried it several times yourself. It is particularly good for people who suffer from insomnia because their minds race and they can't turn off mental energy when they go to bed. Here's how:

Fill a bath with three to four inches of cold water from the tap. Make sure the bathroom is warm and that you have done all of the things you need to do before retiring. Wrap the top half of your body in a sweater or dressing gown which you can tuck up so that when you sit in the water it won't get wet but it will keep the upper part of your body warm. Now immerse your hips and bottom in the tub for 30 seconds. You can do this either by letting your legs hang over the side of the tub or by sitting in the bath and allowing your heels to go into the water to steady your body. Get out, dry yourself well, then climb into bed. The technique draws the body energy away from the head and brings a marvellous sense of peace and relaxation.

Help From the Living Earth

Clay is a pelloid – from the Greek word *pellos* meaning mud. The pelloids are a class of earth substances derived from magma deposits. Amongst natural materials they are unequalled for their therapeutic and health-promoting properties. In Europe they have been used for generations to treat skin, to heal pain and even to deep-cleanse the body by drawing wastes through the skin's surface.

Pelloids are formed in the earth by biological and geological processes over long periods of time – at least 20,000 years. They are made up of both organic and inorganic elements. The 'mostly-organic' pelloids include the sapropelic bituminous muds and the moor or turf pelloids from places like Techirghiol Lake near the Black Sea or Neydharting in Austria. They form the basis of some of the best natural treatments for arthritis, rheumatism, gout and are wonderful for athletic aches and pains as well as for eliminating stiffness from creaky bodies. European scientists at the Institute of Balenology in Bucharest, and in other centres involved in studying the actions of pelloids, have used biochemical, histochemical and clinical methods to examine the effects of the aqueous phase of the moor and turf pelloids and discovered that they can stimulate oxygenation of cells and enzymatic activities in an organism, that they are capable of boosting the endocrine system without interfering with the balance between different glands, and that they dramatically improve overall circulation. Contrary to popular British and American medical beliefs, these extracts appear to penetrate the skin when they are used in a bath or an ointment on the body. Adding them to your bath after a hard game of squash or a long working week in which stress levels have been high can both calm you and regenerate energy levels, as well as improve the look and feel of skin all over the body.

The Seaweed Alternatives

Akin to the actions of the organic pelloids are products based on seaplants and algaes for special 'herbal baths'. They are used primarily for their 'sauna effect' – an ability to cleanse the skin deeply and to eliminate unwanted wastes through the skin. Finely powdered seaweed in bath water helps induce perspiration, increases cell metabolism, tones the skin and soothes aching muscles. The French, who use a lot of the seaplants in this way, claim that the bodily fluids under the skin's surface have a natural affinity with seaweed and on this basis have developed a whole system of seaweed-seawater treatments called thalassotherapy. Certainly the compatibility between seaweed and the body's own blood and lymph chemistry is considerable. Japanese doctors have used extracts of seaweed experimentally to replace blood plasma.

Spring-Cleaning the System with Clay

Best known of pelloids are those which contain mostly inorganic elements – the clays. Therapy using clay, both internally and externally, has a long history. The Egyptians, the Greeks and the Romans all used these earth treatments to improve health, treat athletic aches and sprains and improve the look of skin and hair. Ancient physicians such as the Arab Avicena and Galen the Greek anatomist prescribed clay for patients' ailments. During the First World War Russian soldiers were issued 200 grammes of clay in their food rations, while the French had it added to their mustard because it helps to protect the body from amoebic dysentery which was then so widespread. The great German naturopaths such as Adolph Just used clay to make poultices for wound healing. Recently biologically-oriented French and American doctors have been using certain clays internally as a natural means of detoxifying the body and therefore increasing natural energy levels.

Clay comes in different forms – from kaolin, the pure white powdery stuff that goes into cosmetic products – to the heavy black clay used in the Middle East to treat wounds and bruises. Each has specific qualities and is best for particular purposes. But together they have a number of remarkable things in common. All clays contain a wide range of minerals and trace elements such as silica, magnesium, titanium, iron, calcium, potassium, manganese and chromium. Experts using them claim that these trace elements are important in the dynamic healing actions clays can have on the body. Clay also carries a negative electrical attraction for particles which are positively charged. This is one of the main reasons why it is so good at cleansing both the skin's surface and the digestive tract. Dirt on the surface of the body, like toxic wastes in the system, tends to be positively charged. Dirt particles are drawn to the clay particles with which they come in contact and are then carried away. There are some excellent masks, anti-cellulite products and body wraps for detoxifying the body and enhancing cellular metabolism.

The clays which the French and Americans use for internal cleansing are mixed with water the night before, then taken by mouth on an empty stomach – one teaspoonful in half a glass of water – once a day. These clays are *very* fine. They are made up of minute particles which together have an enormous surface-area-to-volume ratio. Thus they are able to pick up many times their weight in positively-charged particles. In Europe fine green clay is used for this purpose. In America it is usually bentonite – a fine white variety. According to a mineralogist at MIT who has made a particular study of clay, one gramme of bentonite has an extraordinary surface area of 800 square metres. The greater the surface area, the higher a clay's capacity for picking up positively-charged wastes. Ramond Dextreit, a French expert in the use of clay, claims that the purifying capacities of the green clay he uses are not limited to its actions on the digestive system. He says that used in this way it is also able to absorb impurities suspended in body fluids – the blood and lymph for example – and to help drain and eliminate them.

Massage for Calming the Body
Imbalances within the body and disturbances in the internal organs or systems acting through the intervention of related nerves can produce aches and pains, numbness and stiffness in the muscles which in turn can create feelings of discomfort, tenseness and fatigue. Massage is an excellent way of restoring balance and making you feel good again. There are many different forms – from deep tissue massage, acupressure, *shiatsu amma* – the Oriental massage – and lymphatic drainage, to simple stroking of the body. Each has its own benefits. And while some need the trained hands of a professional to be used well, you can bring much benefit to yourself (or a partner) by making simple movements on the surface of the skin with your hands with no training at all. You don't have to know all the right movements. Even 'instinctive massage' can calm hyperactive nerves, relieve stiffness and muscle cramp and make you feel great. There are six basic massage movements:

Effleurage means 'skimming over'. It is a light pressure applied to an area of the body with moving hands. It boosts the circulation of blood and lymph to the areas to which it is being applied, which in turn can improve the functioning of the glands, increase skin sensitivity and heighten the ability of the skin to feel pleasure. Used on your abdomen it can improve the digestive functions of the stomach and intestines and help eliminate constipation. Effleurage also gets rid of chilling sensations in feet or hands when used there, eliminates numbness and decreases any swelling caused by obstructions in the circulatory system.

Begin any massage of yourself or another with effleurage, allowing one hand to follow the other in a rhythmic pattern moving in a direction towards the heart.

Deep Muscle Massage consists of tiny circular movements with a thumb or finger which is firmly pressed into a muscle and then rotated. The finger doesn't actually move over the surface of the skin. Rather it moves the muscle under its pressure. After you have made several small circles in one place you move on to another nearby, always working in an upwards direction on the body. It is excellent for calming overactive nerves and tense muscles and for treating neuralgia or muscular aches. This kind of light pressure on the abdomen improves digestion and elimination. Used in imaginary lines up the limbs it can greatly improve lymphatic drainage and the elimination of wastes.

Single Point Pressure where you press on the surface of the body with the palms, thumbs or fingers, is also good for muscle aches and tensions. It is used when giving acupressure or shiatsu massage for a specific purpose, such as eliminating a headache or calming nerves.

Pétrissage is a kneading movement in which a muscle is held firmly but lightly and moved in circular patterns using the palm of your hand or the balls of your fingers. It increases circulation and is an excellent way of helping muscles recover from fatigue and eliminating lactic acid build-up, which causes muscle ache after a workout. (You need always to keep your fingers relaxed while kneading or you will pinch the skin uncomfortably.)

Vibration is where you put your fingers or palm against the skin of a part of the body and then shake it gently. It is particularly helpful where there is a feeling of numbness – say in fingers or toes.

Tapotement is a tapping with both hands – one after the other – against the skin surface, usually with the palms cupped. It is very invigorating which is why it is always used before sending athletes out on the field but it is not good if you are using massage as a means of 'detensing'.

Putting It All Together

If you are massaging yourself you will need to be in different positions to work on various areas of your body. The legs are easy; they can be done lying on the floor with your legs propped up against the bed or a wall and your head and shoulders against a cushion or two. Or you can simply sit on the edge of a bath. To do your neck and shoulders, it's best to sit at a table with your head lying forward on a pillow in front of you. Lie on your back to do your abdomen and chest and for your lower back, lie on your stomach with a pillow underneath your waist. Then using some oil – vegetable oils are best, simply the kind used to make salads, or you can buy some fine massage oils – begin with an effleurage of the area you are working on and go on to any of the other movements which feel 'right' to you.

Working With A Partner

Use a warm room – usually the floor is best covered with a blanket and a towel. Let your friend or mate lie on his (or her) stomach and begin to work on his back. Never pour cold oil directly onto the skin: instead put it in your hands and give it a chance to warm before applying it. Let him relax as you do an effleurage gently moving up the back, one hand after another. Always maintain contact with his skin so that as one hand is ready to come off the back, the other is already making contact with the skin. And don't be too light or feathery – it makes people feel uneasy; they need to sense good clear contact with your hands to be able to relax deeply. Let him do just that so that he doesn't feel he has to speak if he doesn't want to. Indeed the massage will work better if he doesn't. After you finish a minute or two of effleurage on the back, try a kneading movement or a deep muscle massage on the areas which seem most stiff or uncomfortable. Then, move on to other parts of the body – the feet, the legs, the arms, using the same sequence of movements. Ask him to turn over and work on the front of his legs and arms, the abdomen and the diaphragm. Then finish off with some soothing pétrissage on the shoulders and finally some deeper circular movements to get rid of tension there. End the session with a more gentle effleurage to relax him deeply or do some tapotement to stimulate energy levels, whichever your partner prefers.

The whole process is not as difficult as it may seem if you have never had a go at it. There is quite a wonderful way most people have of finding out how to use these movements, so that they feel good not only to the person being massaged but to yourself. Massage of each other can be an excellent way of communicating for a couple who feel slightly at odds with one another. It eliminates the need for words and seems to restore a sense of unity between people.

Oil Power

Some of the best massage oils are those you mix yourself from a 'carrier oil' such as almond, sesame, coconut, or sunflower, to which you add a small quantity (measured in drops) of specific essential oils – the complex hydrocarbons which give plants and flowers their characteristic odours. Each essential oil has its own biological characteristics and will affect your body in a slightly different way. Depending on what you want from a massage you can choose what is best to use. For instance, four drops each of the essential oils of rosemary, camphor and wintergreen mixed with half a cup of carrier oil makes a superb massage oil for sore muscles after strenuous exercise. Oil of sage mixed with a carrier is good for aches and pains from gardening. A few drops of pure sandalwood or camomile or lavender (or all three together) in a carrier is excellent for relaxing you if you feel tense or under stress. You must make sure that you buy the *real* essential oils however. The chemical analogues which are sometimes sold in their place don't have the same therapeutic effects. These mixtures are also excellent treatments for both male and female skin. They will help keep it moist and protected from the hazards of environmental stress.

The Primitive Brain

The part of the brain which has evolved from the primitive olfactory senses of our animal predecessors is called the lymbic system. It is directly linked to the nose and the pituitary gland – the so-called master gland responsible for the secretion of sex hormones, and concerned with intense emotional drives. This is probably why smells have been known to bring back powerful recollections of events and feelings long ago consciously forgotten.

The lymbic system, in addition to mediating sex drives, hunger, thirst and contentment, appears to be responsible for many of the unusual phenomena of altered states of consciousness: feelings of euphoria, loss of body awareness, sensations of floating or flying and visual sensations such as seeing white or golden light – experiences common to meditation and caused by some drugs.

So the ancients' idea of altering states of consciousness with incense and perfumes is not as superstitious as it once may have seemed.

Fragrance – the Sexual Message

How you smell communicates a great deal to the world around you, particularly in sexual terms. An optimally healthy body gives off subtle odours which convey its vitality. What they are like depends on your own biochemistry and your diet, for each of us has our characteristic smell. Like animals – from the moth to the monkey – we also give off subtle but pervading sexual messages through smell. For many years scientists have been looking at scent communication between species. In the insect world, it is so important that a society of bees or ants could not survive without it – mating, feeding, egg-laying behaviour and social organization are all dependent upon the language of smell. Farmers and vets, too, are well aware of the importance of the odorous chemicals produced by domestic animals. These substances, produced to affect the behaviour or physiology of other animals in specific ways, are called pheromones – a name which was originally coined to describe scent communication between insects, but has come to be used throughout the animal kingdom. Pheromones not only affect overt behaviour, by attracting animals of the opposite sex for mating, for example; they can also profoundly alter the endocrine processes of the animal smelling them.

The latest olfactory research indicates that people also have pheromones (such as androstenol which is found in human sweat and is chemically akin to sex hormones and which – when purified – smells rather like good sandalwood), which send out subliminal messages – many of them sexual – towards others. The effects of the way you smell on someone can be quite dramatic. You can use fragrance to enhance your own enjoyment of an experience or to communicate with others.

Exploring the world of fragrance can be a delightful aesthetic experience. Trying out different fragrances to see how they affect you and the response of others towards you is perhaps the most pleasant of all the body treats and treatments. Don't be misled by masculine and feminine names of perfumes and colognes. There is no such thing as a male or female fragrance. A few years ago women were associated with floral scents and men with woody-spicy ones such as witch hazel, bay, rum and cloves. The direction in perfume now is towards complex blends of wood and spices, musks, florals and aldehydes for both sexes. A so-called men's fragrance can smell wonderful on a woman and many an oriental or rich floral is great on a man. Experiment a little with the different possibilities, ignoring the sex barrier. You might be surprised how much even the fragrances you wear can alter the way you think about yourself and feel in your body.

22
If Only

WHEN MOST PEOPLE think of their body they think of the problems they have with it – or the problems they *think* they have with it. Intermittently plagued by the 'if onlys' – 'if only I didn't have a pot belly . . .', 'if only I weren't so fat . . .', 'if only my eyebrows weren't so bushy . . .' – they are never really satisfied with themselves; but either they don't know how to go about improving what bothers them or they can't summon up the energy to change what can be altered for the better. Almost everybody is in some way dissatisfied with the way their body looks.

Of course chronic dissatisfaction with your looks can signal a deep discomfort of some kind with yourself and have little to do with objective reality. This is why some very attractive people can experience a lot of worry about very minor flaws in 'perfection' while others who are fundamentally far less good-looking exude confidence and feel good about their bodies. The worriers are of the false opinion that 'looks are everything'. Their feelings of self-worth are all wrapped up in the tilt of their nose or the size of their feet. Somewhere along the line they have come to believe that in order to be 'acceptable', 'loved', 'successful', whatever, they have to be perfect.

It's a good notion to throw out if you happen to be one of the 'perfectionists'. The ability to separate your identity and sense of self-worth from the way you look makes it much easier to change the things you don't like about yourself. And really most of these changes are a lot easier to make than you might imagine – provided you want to look great just for the pleasure of it, not because you are totally dependent on it for your sense of self-worth. Start by defining the changes. Then get down to making them. But go easy. . . permanent change usually takes time. Impatience may be one of the worst obstacles you will have to overcome.

If Only I Were Leaner . . .
Excess weight – or rather excess fat – is probably one of the worst psychological stumbling blocks to feeling good about your body. Our society says, 'Fat is ugly . . . anyone who is fat is just weak-willed . . . a second class citizen'. That is all very well for the string beans amongst us. But, anyone who has had to deal with being overweight knows that it is not so easy. Attempts to slim can range from the latest crash diet in a magazine to desperately installing an electronic device which plays the sound of pigs grunting each time you open your refrigerator for an 'illegal' snack. Even the word 'illegal' is a stumbling block to eliminating pounds you don't want and don't need. Most attempts at weight-loss fail because of the assumption that people are fat as a result of being 'weak-willed' or 'cheating' on a diet. You need to look beyond this false assumption and find out what this being 'weak-willed' or 'cheating' is all about. You also need to ask yourself a few questions:

You want to be thinner . . . So what's stopping you?

- 'False hunger' – cravings, bingeing?
- You don't know what is fattening or what a good diet consists of? (See Chapter 8 etc.)
- Don't get enough exercise? (See Chapter 6 etc.)
- Are you psychologically afraid of losing weight? Do you *really* want to be thin?
- Do you like 'bad foods'?

What is False Hunger?
One of the worst obstacles to being thinner is 'false hunger'. It can come in many different forms – cravings for the wrong kinds of foods, or for foods to which you are allergic, a feeling of discomfort after a meal or between meals which makes you want to eat ravenously, or needing energy and reaching for food when you are tired instead of resting or de-stressing with exercise or meditation. Many people have a confusion of messages from stomach to brain

which makes them think they are hungry and need food, although quite the opposite is true. But the discomfort of false hunger is very real. It is the most common reason why someone who places themselves on a slimming regime breaks a diet. No one, not even a 'strong-willed' person, wants to be uncomfortable often or consistently.

False hunger can be the result of many different things. A lot of overweight people, for instance, misread signals from their bodies. If they feel uncomfortable, tired, angry, disappointed or excited, they tend to interpret these feelings as hunger and to think if they have something to eat they will feel better. This keeps them snacking on bits and pieces so that their digestive system never gets a rest – it is in a constant state of stimulation. This is a common reason for false hunger. The more often you eat the more stimulated your digestive system becomes, which in turn produces a renewed feeling of hunger. False hunger can also be the result of food sensitivities or allergies – or cravings for certain foods which seem to be quite irrational. Many people are overweight because they have a hidden allergy to a common food such as wheat, bread or milk. (See page 113.) Food allergies (or, more commonly, sensitivities) are strange things. When you are allergic to something, say milk, and you eat a food which contains it, you are likely to find that you want to eat more and more of that food. Many people who after having one biscuit find they then devour a whole box, are really suffering from a food allergy or sensitivity. When they avoid completely the food to which they are sensitive, the craving and the allergy disappear – so do the extra pounds. Your body chemistry is magic.

Cravings Can Be Clues

If you find you have specific cravings, they can be the result of particular nutritional needs which, because of your own bio-chemical individuality, or the inadequacy of your past diet, have not been satisfied. Here are some of the most common relationships:

● Cola and chocolate, sweets and ice cream – usually people crave them for their caffeine and sugar and for the 'instant energy' lift they will give. Foods rich in B complex vitamins such as liver and wholegrain cereals and breads can help raise energy levels permanently so you don't need a quick boost. So can taking a ten-minute relaxation break where you do a meditation or breathing exercise instead of eating.

● Salty foods – craving salty foods is oftcn a sign of adrenal insuffiency as a result of stress. Many salt-cravers have high blood pressure. If you eliminate salt from your diet completely you will find in a week or two you no longer crave it. Fresh vegetables and grains and pulses have plenty of sodium chloride in them – all your body will ever need. Steer clear of salt.

● Cheese – this can be a sign that you need calcium and phosphorus which is better and more easily available from fresh raw vegetables (lower in calories too).

● Bananas – they are high in potassium. Many people who crave them need more potassium and less sodium – this comes from eating more fresh fruit and vegetables. If you are taking cortisone or diuretics you could need potassium supplements too.

● Apples – good for minerals, these fruits are also a good source of pectin – a form of fibre which lowers cholesterol in the blood and leaches heavy metals such as aluminium from the body. If, in the past, you have eaten a lot of saturated fats your body may need them.

● Nuts – sources of protein, fat or B complex vitamins. You are probably under stress. What can you do about it besides eat?

Awareness is the Key

The key to overcoming false hunger, from whatever cause, is increased awareness of how you feel when it arrives. Once you can identify what is going on, without guilt about being 'weak-willed' – which in truth has nothing to do with it – then you can take steps to change the automatic response of eating more. So when those feelings of hunger arrive after a meal or between meals, STOP. Ask yourself, 'Why am I hungry?'

Have I eaten anything in the last 3 or 4 hours which may have upset my digestion?

Am I tired?

Am I depressed? Angry? Upset?

Do I feel bad about myself or hopeless?

Why do I feel like eating? Is it real hunger or false hunger?

If you discover that you are tired, depressed, anxious or nervous, instead of coping with it as you usually do – by eating something your body doesn't really want or need – look for new ways. Rest. Go for a walk or to a film. Have a conversation with someone about it, or about something completely different. Take a bath. Go for a run or a swim. The sooner you get into the habit of dealing with these feelings in ways other than eating, the quicker your false hunger will disappear.

But I Like 'Bad' Foods

Steering clear of the harmful or energy-depleting foods is nothing more than respecting your body – inside as well as out. Just as you take time every morning to ensure your hair is combed, your body and clothes clean, so you have to care for your insides. And just as you wouldn't want to wear gaudy, garish clothes, when you are aware of what you're doing you won't want to shovel greasy, mushy meals or chocolate bars into your mouth. At first it may seem an austere and maybe impossible step to give up those 'naughty' foods which you so enjoy. Remember though that 'likes' are learnt, so it is a simple matter of gentle re-education to learn to like a new way of eating. People who play the ultrahealth game find that after a few weeks on a good diet, exercising regularly and becoming more aware of their stress patterns and how to cope with them, many junk-food cravings disappear. They no longer want or enjoy the taste of these foods.

Help For That Hideous Appetite

In the meantime there are a few things that can help you if the 'hideous appetite' arrives:

Understand your cravings A good B complex supplement taken three times a day can help to overcome many of them.

Be very organized about eating. Always sit down to eat and put everything you want on to the plate so that the meal ends when you finish and you don't go in for post-meal snacking. Also, don't 'pick' while you are preparing a meal.

Don't eat when you're excited, nervous, over-tired, depressed or angry. In other words make sure your hunger is *real*. If this means missing a meal or two, it won't harm you in the least. Indeed it may help you realize that you don't have to rely on food for energy or comfort.

Get some exercise before a meal. Many of the world's experts in biological medicine recommend that people take exercise, usually in the form of a brisk walk, before each meal. This stimulates your body's metabolic system so that it is more active and able to deal with food more efficiently.

Look out for false hunger first thing in the morning. If you wake ravenously hungry, it is most likely to be false hunger. Ignore it, or have a glass of warm water with lemon and a little honey in it. It will quickly go away. Then mild *real* hunger will follow in an hour or so. It's especially important first thing in the morning not to eat until your system has a chance to wake up and get going.

Don't go to bed on a full stomach. It's best to eat a light evening meal because your body is least active at night. If you eat a heavy meal then it will tend to be deposited as fat stores while you sleep.

Try doing without the occasional meal and drinking some fresh vegetable or fruit juice instead. People have a false notion that if they don't have three good meals a day they are going to faint or feel very ill. In fact, it does you no harm whatsoever to go without a meal when you are not hungry. It gives your digestive system a well-deserved break.

Never use appetite suppressant pills – they are potentially very dangerous to your physical health and to your emotional stability. If you want to try a natural suppressant, and you don't suffer from high blood pressure, consider phenylalanine available from health-food stores. It needs to be taken on an empty stomach in the morning, at least an hour (preferably two) before eating, together with 500 mg of vitamin C and 25 mg of vitamin B6. (See pages 108–9.)

You've probably heard it a hundred times: 'Chew your food well.' In fact, this is one of the most important of all slimming tips. Not only does food fill you up and trigger your satiety mechanism so that you want less when you masticate it fully, the latest research also shows that there is another very important reason for this.

When uncooked fruits and vegetables are chewed well, the enzymes they contain break down into their substrates and form new, health-giving compounds which not only make you feel satisfied but can also improve overall wellbeing.

Tricks and Treatments for Special Areas of the Body

Another constant source of concern to many men and women are specific areas of their body which don't look the way they would like because muscles are slack and out of condition or because there is too much flab. While it is true that there are some excellent movements you can do to help these things, it is even more true that when you get yourself into an ultrahealth way of living you will find many of these long-term 'problems' seem rather mysteriously to vanish. The best kind of exercise for a spreading waistline is 40 minutes of an aerobic activity about 5 or 6 times a week. The foods you eat also influence the state of your flesh and muscles. A year on fresh natural foods, many of them raw without refined sugar, with little fat and not too much protein, will completely renew the look of your body all over. In the meantime, however, it can be very useful to do a little work, say before a bath every day, on areas that need special attention. Remember that to get results you need to be consistent in your efforts – do only the ones you feel you need, but make sure it is every day. Here are the most common body problems and some solutions:

For Men
The Problem: Pot Belly

Give up eating refined carbohydrates such as foods made from white sugar and/or white flour and stop drinking beer.

Do the Abdominal Hold while sitting at a desk, standing against a wall or waiting in traffic:

Sitting or standing erect, suck in your stomach as hard as you can with your abdominal muscles so that it feels as though your stomach is pressing against your backbone. Hold for six seconds then relax and repeat about a dozen times. Talk and breathe normally while doing the exercise. You can repeat this several times a day.

Practise Half Sit-Ups: Lie on the floor with your knees bent, hands behind your head. Keeping chin against chest, roll your torso up so your head is only 8–10 inches off the floor, and with your lower back pressed firmly against the floor, hold there for a slow count of three. Then roll slowly back down and relax. Repeat up to 30 times.

The Problem: Hunched, Tense Shoulders

Every time you find yourself getting tense, with your shoulders hunched up towards your ears, consciously pull them downwards. It is an amazingly 'freeing' feeling and even helps you think more clearly. There are also some very good movements specifically to improve joint movement in the shoulders which you should do at least once a day (each movement):

Standing with your back against a wall, arch your back in exaggeration for a moment, thrusting your shoulders back, and then curve it, as though you were bringing together your two shoulders at the front. Do this in a rhythmic movement 20 times.

Sitting or standing straight, allowing your arms to hang free, without bending your arms or moving shoulders back, lift your shoulders towards your ears. Now, gently and slowly lower them, lengthening your neck.

Sit or stand upright with feet slightly apart. Let your arms hang loose and relaxed at your sides. With your neck relaxed move your shoulders forward, up, back and down in a circle, making a continuous motion. Repeat six times in each direction.

These movements will also help an underdeveloped or sunken chest.

The Problem: Poor Posture

This is one of the most common 'flaws' in otherwise attractive men. To have good posture you need first to know what it feels like. You also need to have good muscle strength in your abdominals and back, so exercises designed for them can be helpful. The best thing possible is to study the Alexander Technique if you can find a good teacher. Next best is practising the pelvic lift against a wall.

Hands on your hips, heels two inches from the wall, with your head, shoulders, elbows and buttocks against the wall, pull in your stomach and tighten your buttocks while gently rotating your pelvis forward until the curve of your lower spine flattens against the wall. (You will have to bend your knees slightly to do this and you can use your hands to get the feel of the pelvis tipping until you get used to the sensation.) Tilt it slowly backwards and forwards ten times. Then, holding the position, gently slide down the wall a foot or two all the while keeping your lower back, head, shoulders and elbows pressed against it. Now, gently come back up again, trying to keep all of these parts still pressed against the wall. You will sense a pulling on your lower back muscles throughout this exercise which can be done several times a day, just before you go into a meeting, when you get up in the morning, before you go to bed at night. It helps give you the feel of what good posture is like. Do it often enough so you know, and then try reproducing this feel while you are walking around or standing and sitting until it becomes quite easy.

For Women
The Problem: Thick or Heavy Thighs
Change the way you are eating to include lots of fresh raw vegetables so that you encourage detoxification of your system. (The Biogenic Clean-Up is excellent to start you off.) If you have cellulite it is an internal pollution problem. It has to be treated from within and without all at once to banish it once and for all.

Do skin brushing twice a day, morning and night (see page 254).

Lying on your side with your body slightly curved and supported on an elbow with the other hand in front of you for balance, raise both legs so that the one underneath is about 2 inches off the floor. Then, keeping them raised, swing them back and forth as if you were doing a goose step, never swinging the back leg beyond the hip. Start with 10 times and work up to 25 times, then change sides and repeat.

Lying on your side with your head on one arm outstretched beneath it, put the other hand in front of you for support and bend your underneath leg. Keeping the top leg straight, raise it, with toes pointing as far upwards as you can. Then lower slowly to the floor. Start with 10 times and work up to 25. Change sides and repeat. This is also good for the sides of the hips, your calves and your arches.

Using a tennis ball or any small ball you have available, lie on your back with your knees bent and your feet together on the floor. Put the ball between your knees. You may need to stretch out your arms above your head and steady yourself by holding on to the legs of a heavy chair. Now, slowly, squeeze the ball together with your thighs and, leaving your back flat on the floor, bring both thighs all the way over to the right and then all the way over to the left without allowing the ball to drop. Do this 10 times to each side. (This exercise is also good for the waist and back.)

Take up weight training with a good teacher using free weights.

The Problem: Sagging Breasts

Every morning take a shower in hot water then, when your body is well warmed, switch to cold and direct the spray on your breasts for thirty seconds. (You can start with 10 seconds and work up.)

Smiling, exaggerate the movement into a grimace so that the muscles in your neck become contracted. Hold for five seconds and repeat 20 times. This is good for the neck as well as the bust.

Putting your hands together in front of you in a 'praying position' with palms together, push your elbows upwards and lift fingertips to the height of your chin. Now push your palms together as hard as you can for three seconds. Repeat 20 times breathing deeply all the while. Then grasp your fingers in a hook shape with the fingers of the opposite hand and pull hard for three seconds, again breathing deeply. Repeat 20 times.

Try the 'posture correctors' in the men's section. A lot of bust problems come from bad posture.

For Men and Women
The Problem: Spreading Waistline

Do some butterfly kicks. Lying on your back on the floor, feet together, raise them 10 inches off the floor and then move them as if you were swimming the crawl, one after the other. Do this 20 times. Relax for a moment and then repeat twice more.

In the same position, raise your legs off the floor and this time do small scissor kicks, crossing and beating your calves together in three sets of ten beats each.

Lying on your back with your torso raised off the floor and supported on your elbows, keeping both legs together raise them so they are at a 90 degree angle to the floor and flex your feet. Now, trying to flatten your stomach and exhaling, bring your legs slowly down to the floor. Then, bend your knees, drawing your heels towards your buttocks, raise your feet off the ground and straighten your legs in the air again. Repeat 10 times, rhythmically breathing in as you raise your legs and out as you lower them.

Lying on your side on the floor with your head on an arm stretched out beneath it and the lower leg bent underneath you, foot flexed, raise your top leg up and then bring it down again 15 times. Do three sets of 15.

Standing tall, with your feet shoulder distance apart, reach up as high as you can with your hands above your head. Now stretch high all along one side of your body with your arm, bending the leg on the same side to increase the stretch. Then switch to the other arm changing rhythmically from one to the other. Do three sets of 10.

The Problem: Double Chin
Lying on a bed on your back with your head hanging over the edge, slowly open your mouth and close it 15 times. Rest for a moment then do two more series of 30.

Sitting upright or standing, tilt your head back so your face is parallel to the ceiling. Now open your mouth and stick out your tongue tilting it downwards as far as it will go. Now return your head to normal position. Repeat six times, rest for a moment and do two more series of six.

In the same position, tilt your head back so your face is parallel with the ceiling, then stick out your lower jaw and bring it back in again as you lower your head to normal. Repeat three times. Do three series of three.

The Problem: Rough Skin
Give yourself a salt rub before your bath or shower. Here's how: take a small bowl of rough sea salt and dampen it so that it tends to clump together. Using a handful of the salt, rub it all over your damp body with a scrubbing motion. Then shower it off and apply a natural oil such as sesame, almond, coconut or a massage oil (see page 260).

Consider taking supplements of GLA and lecithin (one table-spoon of granular lecithin sprinkled into juice, yogurt or over salad). (See pages 108–9.)

Make a comfrey compress for any area which is severely dried out or flaky such as hands or face. Comfrey is probably the most useful herb of all for helping skin which is rough, irritated or blotched. Make a compress by pouring half a cup of boiling water over a handful of the dried herb: let it cool to a bearable temperature, then put the wet herb on a layer of gauze which you have placed over your face, or wherever, and cover it with more gauze. Rest for 15 minutes while it takes effect and cools. This kind of compress will also reduce the pain and swelling of a bruise or a pulled muscle.

The Problem: Body Odour and Bad Breath

Have your zinc and manganese levels checked and if low, take zinc and manganese supplements which act as 'internal deodorants' in doses of 25–50 mg of the chelated minerals a day.

For breath problems, make sure you brush your teeth carefully and long twice a day and floss once a day. Peridontal disease is the most common cause of bad breath if your body is otherwise well.

The Problem: Varicose Veins

Elevate your legs at every opportunity. This drains stagnant blood from areas with poor circulation and brings fresh blood in. Whenever you can, use a slantboard. It is not only good for varicose veins but for skin and for relaxation as well. And it is easy to make one. You need a plank wide enough to take the width of your body and a foot or two longer than you are, raised at one end by fifteen inches. Lie on it head-down-feet-up for a few minutes each day. It reverses the pull of gravity on your body and is deeply refreshing. Your facial muscles get pulled up instead of down, pressure is taken off the legs and feet and the vascular system and you will get up feeling renewed and refreshed. Try it while you are listening to music (preferably of the serene and melodic kind!) for the most wonderful sensation of overall relaxation. Start with 15 minutes a day and work up to 30.

Also, try to remember to apply cold water to your legs after *any* hot water (bath, shower, etc.). Don't strain your legs unnecessarily, don't wear tight-waisted clothes, and make arrangements to elevate the foot of your bed permanently by three to four inches.

Consider taking 400 to 800 IU of vitamin E each day – 200 to 400 in the morning and 200 to 400 at night. Vitamin E is excellent for circulatory problems. The Canadian expert on the vitamin, Dr. Evan Shute, reassures people who use this treatment that they can occasionally get pain in their legs just after beginning the therapy, which is a sign that new capillaries are forming. If it is too uncomfortable, he says, you should reduce the dosage and then gradually build up again. If you have high blood pressure it is important to start with only small quantities of vitamin E – 50–100 IU and then gradually increase the amount you are taking. Other nutrients which are said to be helpful for varicose veins include the bioflavonoids – particularly rutin – 100–200 mg a day; Vitamin C – 1,500–4,000 mg a day; pantothenic acid (Vitamin B5) – 50–150 mg a day; and calcium – 500–1,000 mg a day.

The Problem: Weak, Soft, or Splitting Nails

Look to your diet. If you have tiny white flecks on your nails, this can be a sign of zinc or silicon deficiency. They can usually be corrected in a few weeks by taking 25 to 50 mg of chelated zinc or zinc orotate daily. Consider taking organic silicon derived from the horsetail plant at meals.

If your nails are brittle and break easily you might try brewer's yeast tablets – six with each meal or, better still, stirring a teaspoon to a tablespoon of powdered brewer's yeast into a glass of juice two times a day and taking two kelp tablets with each meal.

If you are plagued by hangnails, try puncturing a 200 IU capsule of vitamin E and rubbing it around the base of your nails every evening.

The Problem: Easy Bruising or Fine Broken Veins

Try supplements of vitamin C together with the bioflavonoids –500 mg of each three times a day plus 25–50 mg of chelated zinc or zinc picolinate.

Stay away from extremes of temperature on your skin and protect your face when you are out in winter with a rich moisturizer or an oil.

The Problem: Excess Body Hair

For women's legs, remove hair by shaving or waxing or using a depilatory. Shaving is the easiest way but you get the greatest regrowth with it. Waxing can be painful but regrowth is slower. A depilatory can be very irritating to skin unless you have very strong skin.

For permanent hair removal for either a man or a woman you need to use epilation or electrolysis. Epilation removes hair by short-wave diathermy (heat), which coagulates the root of the hair and the cells surrounding it and eventually destroys the ability of the follicle to produce a hair. Electrolysis removes hair by galvanic means; chemical substances formed at the tip of the needle destroy the hair root. Both methods are carried out with the use of a very fine needle which has to be put into the hair follicle individually. It is a slow (and sometimes painful) process but permanent. It can be an excellent way of removing unwanted hair from the face, such as thinning out the brows of a man which have grown together over the nose or removing hair on the upper lip of a woman. It needs to be done by a well-trained operator.

Ask a Friend or Three

All of these exercises, treatments and nutritional approaches can be helpful in solving specific body problems which make you feel less than good about yourself. What they can't do, however, is alter the belief that you are unattractive if it comes from poor self-esteem. For that you need help from regular exercise and the changes in brain chemistry which it brings about; also from some of the things in the Mind Games section (see Part Five).

Something that can be very reassuring if there is some feature you dislike about yourself or some aspect of your body you can't come to terms with is this: ask three good friends to list two negative and two positive things about the way you look. (This is an excellent way to test out just how much of a problem some particular 'flaw' is.) Then compare their answers with your own evaluation. You are likely to find that the things which bother you most are often not even noticed by others, and discover several positive aspects of your body and your looks that you may not now appreciate. It helps put things in perspective. Keeping everything in perspective is absolutely essential to developing any lifestyle for ultrahealth. A lot of self-conscious flaws seem to disappear by magic when you manage to do this

PART EIGHT

GET IT TOGETHER

23
Take Control

SO THAT'S THE story. You've looked at the six dimensions of ultrahealth – nutritional action, physical fitness, stress management, self-responsibility, age control and environmental awareness. You've examined some of the obstacles in playing the ultrahealth game – such as life in the twentieth century, social norms which encourage worseness rather than wellness, and the ravages of Kronos – and hopefully had a glimpse of what, by involving yourself in the ultrahealth play, can be possible for you in terms of increased energy, good looks and high-level wellness. If you like what you've seen, then only one thing remains: getting down to business to make as many of the ultrahealth payoffs part of your own life as you can. There are a couple of things which can help a lot.

Learning the vital signs. Becoming familiar with the measurements, both objective and subjective, which can tell you now or at any time in the future just how far and how fast you are progressing in your ultrahealth play.

Outlining a Personal Ultrahealth Plan

Measuring the Changes
Having some gauge of your progress towards ultrahealth can not only reassure you that what you are doing for yourself is right, it can also give you the motivation to continue whenever the tendency to collapse in a heap and go back to worseness-oriented ways suddenly appears. It is useful to have objective measurements. The problem

is that our medical system, while it has developed superb tests for measuring your state of ill health, knows almost nothing about measuring wellness. Modern medical procedures such as laboratory tests for cholesterol and triglyceride levels in the blood, as well as measurements of blood pressure, resting heart-rate and the vital capacity of the lungs can be helpful to some degree. If you have a physical examination now testing these things, then follow an ultrahealth lifestyle for six months and have them tested again, you will certainly find that they have improved greatly. But there is a catch here too. A lot of what is considered 'normal' in terms of blood pressure, heart-rate, cholesterol levels and so forth according to orthodox medicine is probably nothing of the kind. The 'norms' by which you are measured have been established by testing 'unsick' people and comparing 'averages'. So far there are no measurements available of *ultrahealthy* people to which you can compare yourself. For instance, the average doctor considers someone's heart-rate 'normal' if it's 90 beats a minute. But people who are truly fit and who live on a low-fat diet high in fresh raw foods tend to have heart-rates down in the 40s, 50s and 60s. A similar situation exists in measuring blood pressure and vital capacity. So by all means have these tests done now and then in six months and compare. You'll be delighted with the results. But don't think that, because your doctor congratulates you on being 'in the best of health', that you necessarily are – yet. If you want to achieve high-level wellness you are going to have to take most 'normal' parameters of measurement with a grain of salt. They are simply not good enough.

The Progress Check List
Nonetheless tests can be useful and – particularly at the beginning of ultrahealth play – fun to take. Here is a short list of some of the parameters which can be measured.

Resting Heart-Rate: This tells you about the state of your cardiovascular resistance – in other words the strength of your heart and how efficient your blood circulation is. It is best done by taking your pulse first thing in the morning when you are lying in bed. As you become fitter your heart-rate decreases so that instead of, say, having to beat 80 times a minute to pump the blood around your body, it only has to beat 50 times. Resting pulse decreases significantly after about six months on a regular aerobic exercise programme. Taking your resting heart-rate (see pages 65–6) now, and then comparing it in a few months' time, will give you an objective indication of your increasing condition.

Heart Recovery Rate: How fast your heart-rate returns to normal after exercise is another measurement of fitness. (See pages 59–60.) This rate too will decrease significantly and is an excellent benchmark of your progress.

Percentage of Body Fat: The bulk of your body mass is made up of two kinds of tissue – muscle and fat. The ultrahealthy person, unlike the average Briton or American with his tendency to be overweight (20–25 per cent fat is 'normal' for men and 24–27 per cent for women) has a remarkably low percentage of body fat – 15 per cent or less for men and 18 per cent or less for women. This can be accurately measured using a hydrostatic tank where your body is immersed in a tub of warm water and then weighed under water or by an electrical impedance unit such as the Bodystat. The weight recorded is compared with your body weight. The more you weigh under water, the less body fat you are carrying. Another slightly less accurate but still adequate way of measuring body weight is with skin-fold calipers which you can buy yourself. They measure the thickness of a pinch of skin at the back of the upper arm, the waist and other areas and then refer you to tables by which you can interpret the total percentage of fat in your body. This measurement can be very helpful in monitoring your progress in the ultrahealth game.

Pulmonary Function Tests: There are several ways of measuring how well your body uses oxygen: in other words, your respiratory efficiency and your vital capacity. By using a peak flowmeter which you breathe into, a doctor, nurse or physiotherapist can find out how well you take up oxygen in the air to make use of it in your body, how well that oxygen is transferred to your blood and a lot about the elasticity of your lungs and breathing tubes. Although not always readily available, and although such tests are medically controlled, this is a very good measurement for the ultrahealth player wanting to check his progress. It can however take longer here to see results – try having pulmonary function tests done now, if possible, and then in a year or even two.

Self-Monitoring Starts Here

Even more important, I think, is the kind of self-monitoring you do on your own. Unfortunately, unlike the vital measurements listed above, it is not objective. It depends on your own subjective judgements about how you feel and how you're changing. But to me, these are the most valuable measurements of all because they are part of a personal feedback system which, once you get into the feel of it, is extraordinarily reliable. Here are a few examples of self-monitoring questions. Answer them and make notes of them in a journal. Then compare your answers with the way you answer in six weeks' time, three months' time, six months' time and so forth:

How well do you sleep? Do you need a lot of sleep or are you content with six or seven hours a night? Do you dream vividly? Do your dreams seem of interest to you and do they have meaning? Or do you simply 'crash out' when you hit the bed each night?

How do you feel when you get up in the morning? Clear-headed and cheerful? Looking forward to the day ahead no matter what it brings? Or are you still fatigued after a night's sleep? Would you prefer to stay in bed for the rest of the morning if you could?

How are your energy levels throughout the day? Do you feel you need a cup of coffee to keep going? Do you have a tendency to 'wear out' in the middle of the afternoon? Are you bouncy enough after a day's work that you can look forward to going out in the evening?

How much fun do you have? Do you find yourself laughing easily at little things? Are you able to enjoy yourself without heavy doses of alcohol and being entertained all the time? Do you enjoy your work as much as your play?

How good do you look? Is your skin clear, your hair strong and shiny and are your nails strong? How do you feel about your looks? Are you pleased, even though there may be a few things you'd change?

How do you feel about your life? Is it something you only endure or something you feel quite excited about, particularly when you look towards the future? Would you trade places with anybody else in the world?

It is important that you record your answers to these questions honestly and as accurately as you can in a journal or notebook which is kept for your eyes only. If you simply answer verbally you won't get much from the experience. You need black and white evidence made today in front of you which you can then compare with your answers to the same questions in a few weeks' or months' time. It will give you an excellent sense of the progress you are making.

In fact, a journal or diary tucked away in a drawer for you to refer to and record things in is one of the best tools for playing the ultrahealth game you will find. It is particularly helpful for working out a good strategy for your ultrahealth play and for making real progress. After you have answered the questions above, taken a few of the vital measurements and recorded the 'statistics' in your diary, you're ready to start planning.

Working Out a Personal Plan
The better organized and more definite a plan you make for yourself, the more you will benefit from the material in this book. Such a plan should set out your commitments and clarify your intentions. It will help you make the best use of your resources within the context of your work and private life. It will also stress your own sense of responsibility about the changes you will be making. In effect, a definite plan helps you to take seriously what you are doing. It can also be a source of considerable personal insight.

Be Specific
The more specific your preliminary plan, the better. Pick one goal for ultrahealth which interests you particularly now – say becoming more physically fit or learning better methods of stress control, or losing weight. Make a plan for yourself with specific goals such as: 'I intend in a month to have 6 pounds less fat on my body.' It is no good to say 'I intend to lose weight.' That is far too vague to provide a potent impetus for change. Then plan how to go about it – on

paper. Ask yourself what ultrahealth tools you might use to reach your goal. Here are a few suggestions:

I'll use *The Biogenic Clean-Up* for ten days beginning next Friday to get me started. (See page 82.)

I'll begin an exercise programme of *rebounding* (see page 62) tomorrow. (This commitment entails a corollary – that of organizing the buying of a rebounder today, to be ready for tomorrow. If this doesn't seem possible, you'll have to postpone your intention until, say, next week when it is. If a rebounder is too expensive then you will have to alter your exercise plan to fit in with the possibilities, say by going swimming three times a week or beginning to jog or going for brisk walks three times a week instead.)

There is always the chance I may be hungry at first until my appetite adjusts to the new way of eating. I will therefore buy some phenylalanine (see page 268), vitamin B6 and vitamin C to take as nutritional supplements in the morning – just to have them on hand if I do.

I might need to learn a couple of useful *destressing exercises* (page 159) to help me deal with tensions instead of turning to food as I usually do. I will begin on that today.

Such a preliminary plan will get you going very clearly with a good sense of direction and a knowledge of just what you will have to do in specific terms to reach your goal.

Record Your Impressions
As you go along, it's helpful to write down things which happen, obstacles which get in your way and how you might solve (or have solved) them. For instance, some obstacles might be:

● My husband *hates* salads and has to have his coffee after every meal,
or
● The people in my office might make fun of me if I take up an exercise programme,

or
- I've tried to lose weight before and I've always failed,

or
- My wife might resent my taking meal planning into my own hands.

If you get all the possible obstacles you can think of down on paper you can then look for ways of getting round them. (In fact, one of the most useful ways around many is to involve other people in what you are doing. A lot of lounge lizards would secretly like to be dynamically fit and slim too, they are just too shy to say so – or too afraid to 'go for it' lest they 'fail'.)

Structure Your Day

This is important. And this too can be worked out in your notebook. It is no good planning to do 30 minutes of rebounding and drink juice for breakfast if you have no juice extractor and you don't know when you are going to find time for the rebounding. You need to work out a specific plan. Then test it out and change it when you find a better way of doing things or as you change. There is absolutely no reason why any ultrahealth lifestyle should take away from the other things in your day. It is a matter of managing time well.

One of the wonderful things about playing the ultrahealth game is that the longer you play, the more time you find you have available to you for other things. For instance, eating the ultrahealth way you detoxify your system of stored wastes which have been depleting your energy and by doing so, you create more energy for work and play. Regular exercise can also bring increased energy for other activities. So the hours you spend working are more efficient and enjoyable and the time you take out for your exercise programme becomes insignificant besides the benefits in terms of efficiency during the rest of your day.

Eating lots of raw vegetables and no refined foods means that you will probably want to sleep less too. That has happened to nearly everyone I know who has gone over to the ultrahealth way of eating. On these foods your body seems to need less time in the night to repair its tissues and to detoxify.

Sample Plan

To give you some idea of what a day's plan might be, I will show you my own – not that it is any paragon of efficiency, and it certainly won't be the way I am living six months from now. It will change as I change. But for the moment it works for me:

Ultrahealth Schedule

5.15	Get up
5.30–5.50	Meditation and prayers
5.50–6.05	*Skin Brushing* (page 254)
	Shower and *Cold Shower* (page 254)
	Quick Rub Down with Massage Oil (page 260)
	Dress
6.05	Go to my studio to work until 8.00
8.00–9.00	Make *Raw Juice* (page 91) for the day and have breakfast
9.00–12.30	Work
12.30–2.00	Lunch and rest with *Autogenic Training* (page 159)
2.00–5.30	Work
5.30–6.30	Weight training 1–1½ hours every other day, plus ½ hour running or rowing on alternate days.
6.30–7.00	Shower and Dress
7.00	onwards – free for the evening
11.30	Ready for bed. *Autogenic Training* again
11.35	Sleep

Your daily plan will look very different from mine. Indeed my own is different when I am working in London or travelling, instead of at home writing. What matters is to find a way in which you can fit in all of the things you want to do for yourself with the demands of your work and the needs of the other people you live and work with. And whatever plan you make, expect it to change as you do. Both will.

Make Notes of Your Successes

Write down as you go along the successes you have – the time it takes you to run your two miles and how it is improving, the loss of another pound, the look of your skin that causes someone to comment, 'You look great!' They can be a pleasure and a help to refer to when you find yourself on one of those weight-loss 'plateaux' which you just have to ride out before things start happening again. Then every three months re-evaluate your plan and restructure it. As you gain in fitness and wellness even your goals change.

Ultrahealth Becomes Easy

In time you will find that the ultrahealth way of life becomes second nature to you. What at first may have seemed an effort – such as giving up your six cups of coffee, or putting on those running shoes and getting out on the road – now becomes a pleasure and so much a natural part of your life that you won't even have to give it a thought.

Instead of having to resist eating that chocolate bar which you've always thought you couldn't do without, you will wonder why you ever wanted it. You will come to believe that looking good and feeling great is 'normal' and you will love it. At that point, playing the ultrahealth game becomes a source of real fun and you can forget all about the 'rules'. You will have become a Master.

Further Reading

Part One: Ultrahealth vs 20th Century Life

The Berkeley Holistic Health Handbook: A Tool for Attaining Wholeness of Body, Mind and Spirit Berkeley, Calif.: And/Or Publishers, 1978.

BOHM, D. *Wholeness and the Implicate Order* London: Routledge and Kegan Paul, 1980.

CARLSON, Rick. *The End of Medicine* New York: Wiley, 1975.

DAVIS, Steven Andrew, MD. *How To Stay Healthy in a Polluted World* New York: William Morrow & Company Inc., 1983.

DOSSEY, Larry, MD. *Space, Time & Medicine* London: Shambhala, 1982.

EISEMBERG, L. 'What Makes Persons "Patients" and "Patients" Well?' *American Journal of Medicine* 69: 277–286, 1980.

ENGLE, George L. 'The Need for a New Medical Model: A Challenge For Biomedicine', *Science* 196, 1977, pp. 129–136.

ILLICH, I. *Medical Nemesis – The Expropriation of Health* New York: Pantheon, 1976.

LALONDE, Marc. *A New Perspective on the Health of Canadians* Ottawa: Government of Canada, 1974.

PELLETIER, Kenneth. *Holistic Medicine* New York: Delacorte Press/ Seymour Lawrence, 1979.

PELLETIER, Kenneth. *Toward a Science of Consciousness* New York: Delacorte Press, 1978.

ROBERTS, Toni M., Tinker, Kathleen, and Kemper, Donald W. *Healthwise Handbook: A Guide to Responsible Health Care* Garden City, NY: Doubleday, 1979.

SURGEON GENERAL, The. *Healthy People: The Surgeon General's Report on Health Promotion and Disease Prevention* DHEW, Pubs Nos 79–55071 and 79–55071A: Washington, DC: 1979.

WALDBOTT, G. L. *Health Effects of Environmental Pollutants* St Louis: Mosby, 1973.

Part Two: Body Power

BAILEY, Covert. *Fit or Fat* New York: Houghton-Mifflin, 1978.

BALASKAS, Arthur, and Janet. *New Life* London: Sidgwick & Jackson, 1979.

BALASKAS, Arthur and Stirk, John. *Soft Exercise* London: Unwin Paperbacks, 1983.

COOPER, Kenneth H. *The New Aerobics* New York: Bantam, 1970.

DE VRIES, Herbert. *Health Science: A Positive Approach* Santa Monica, Calif.: Goodyear, 1979.

FIXX, James. *The Complete Book of Running* London: Chatto and Windus, 1979.

KENNEDY, Pat. *The Moving Body* London: Faber and Faber, 1979.

KENTON, Leslie. *Lean Revolution* London: Random House, 1994.

KUNTZLEMAN, Charles T. *Activetics* New York: Wyden, 1978.

MIRKIN, Gabe, MD, and Hoffman, Marshall. *The Sportsmedicine Book* Boston: Little, Brown and Company, 1978.

MOOREHOUSE, L. *The Physiology of Exercise* 7th edn. St. Louis: Mosby, 1976.

NEWTON-DONN, Esme. *The Bodywork Book* London: Collins, 1982.

NOBLE, Elizabeth. *Essential Exercises for the Childbearing Year* London: John Murray, 1978.

SHEEHAN, George. *Dr. Sheehan on Running* Mountain View, Calif.: World, 1975.

SPENO, Dyveke. *New Age Training for Fitness and Health* New York: Grove Press, 1979.

Part Three: High-Energy Nutrition

BIRCHER, Ralph ed. *Dr. Bircher-Benner's Way to Positive Health and Vitality* Zürich: Bircher-Benner Verlag, 1976.

BIRCHER-BENNER CLINIC, *Bircher-Benner Raw Food and Juices Nutrition Plan* Los Angeles: Nash, 1973.

BRONFEN, Nan. *Nutrition For A Better Life* Santa Barbara, Calif.: Capra Press, 1980.

COLGAN, Michael. *Your Personal Vitamin Profile* London: Blond and Briggs, 1983.

KENTON, Leslie, and Kenton, Susannah. *Raw Energy* London: Century, 1993.

PFEIFFER, Carl C., and Banks, Jane. *Dr Pfeiffer's Total Nutrition* New York: Simon and Schuster, 1980.

PFEIFFER, Carl C., MD. *Mental and Elemental Nutrients* New Canaan, Conn: Keats, 1975.

PRITIKIN, Nathan. *The Pritikin Programme for Diet and Exercise* New York: Grosset and Dunlap, 1979.

SCHWARTZ, George, MD. *Food Power* New York: McGraw-Hill, 1979.

SZÉKELY, Edmond Bordeaux. *Guide To The Essene Way of Biogenic Living* Cartago, Costa Rica: International Biogenic Society, 1977.

SZÉKELY, Edmond Bordeaux. *The Book of Living Foods* Cartago, Costa Rica: International Biogenic Society, 1977.

WILLIAMS, Roger J. *Nutrition in a Nutshell* New York: Dolphin Books, 1962.

WILLIAMS, Roger J. *Physicians' Handbook of Nutritional Science* Springfield: Charles C. Thomas, 1978.

WILLIAMS, Roger J., and Kalits, Dwight K. eds *A Physician's Handbook of Orthomolecular Medicine* New Canaan, Conn.: Keats, 1977.

WILSON, Frank. *Successful Sprouting* Wellingborough: Thorsons, 1978.

Part Four: Mind Games

ALBRIGHT, Peter and Bets, eds. *Mind, Body and Spirit* Findhorn, Scotland: Thule Press, 1980.

BROWN, Barbara. *Supermind* New York: Bantam Books, 1983.

DYCHTWALD, Ken. *Bodymind* London: Wildwood, 1978.

FINK, D. H. *Release From Nervous Tension* London: Unwin Paperbacks, 1979.

GOLDWAG, Eliott. *Inner Balance – The Power of Holistic Healing* Englewood Cliffs, NJ: Prentice-Hall, 1979.

JACOBSON, Edmund, MD. *You Must Relax* London: Souvenir, 1977.

KENTON, Leslie. *The New Joy of Beauty* London: Vermilion, 1995.

LIEBERMAN, Harris R., Wurtman, Richard J. eds. *Research Strategies for Assessing The Behavioral Effects of Foods and Nutrients* Proceedings of a Conference held at the Massachusetts Institute of Technology, Cambridge, Mass. on November 9, 1982: Center for Brain Sciences and Metabolism Charitable Trust.

MADDERS, Jane. *Stress and Relaxation* London: Martin Dunitz, 1979.

MASLOW, A. H. *The Farther Reaches of Human Nature* New York: The Viking Press, 1975.

MASON, L. John. *Guide to Stress Reduction* Culver City, Calif.: Peace Press, 1980.

MEARNES, Ainslie, MD. *Relief Without Drugs* London: Fontana, 1967.

NARANJO, Claudio, and Ornstein, Robert. *On the Psychology of Meditation* New York: Penguin, 1972.

NEWBOLD, H. L. *Mega-Nutrients For Your Nerves* New York: Peter H. Wyden, 1975.

OYLE, Irving. *Time, Space and the Mind* Milbrae, Calif.: Celestial Arts, 1976.

PEARCE, Joseph Chilton. *Magical Child* London: Paladin, 1979.

PEARCE, Joseph Chilton. *The Bond of Power* London: Routledge and Kegan Paul, 1982.

PELLETIER, Kenneth. *Mind as Healer, Mind as Slayer: A Holistic Approach to Preventing Stress Disorders* New York: Delacorte and Delta, 1977.

PELLETIER, Kenneth. *Toward a Science of Consciousness* New York: Delacorte Press, 1978.

ROGERS, Carl. *On Becoming a Person* London: Constable, 1977.

SELYE, Hans. *Stress Without Distress* London: Hodder and Stoughton, 1974.

SELYE, Hans. *The Stress of Life*. New York: McGraw-Hill, 1976.

SHEALY, Norman C., MD. *90 Days to Self-Health*, New York: Dial Press, 1977.

WEINBERG, George. *Self Creation* London: Macdonald and Jane's, 1978.

Part Five: Ageless Ageing

ABBOT, David. *New Life For Old – Therapeutic Immunology* London: Frederick Muller, 1981.

BENET, Sula. *How to Live to Be 100: The Lifestyle of the People of the Caucasus* New York: Dial Press, 1976.

CURTIN, Sharon R. *Nobody Ever Died of Old Age* Boston: Little, Brown and Co., 1972.

DUBOS, Rene. *A God Within* New York: Charles Scribner's, 1972.

FRANK, Benjamin. *Dr. Frank's No-Ageing Diet* New York: Dell, 1976.

FRANKLIN, Olga. *H3* London: Arthur Barker, 1964.

KENT, Saul. *The Life Extension Revolution* New York: Quill, 1983.

KENTON, Leslie. *The New Ageless Ageing* London: Vermilion, 1995.

KUGLER, Hans J. *Slowing Down the Ageing Process* New York: Pyramid, 1974.

KUGLER, Hans. *Doctor Kugler's Seven Keys to a Longer Life* New York: Fawcett Crest, 1978.

LAMB, Marion J. *Biology of Ageing* London: Blackie, 1977.

LINDSAY, Rae. *The Pursuit of Youth* New York: Pinnacle, 1976.

LUMIÈRE, Cornel. *The Fountain of Youth* Geneva: Editions du Mont-Blanc, 1971.

PASSWATER, Richard. *Supernutrition – Mega-vitamin Revolution* New York: Pocket Book, 1977.

PEARSON, Dirk, and Shaw, Sandy. *Life Extension – A Practical Scientific Approach* New York: Warner, 1982.

PELLETIER, Kenneth R. *Longevity – Fulfilling Our Biological Potential* New York: Delacorte Press/Seymour Lawrence, 1981.

ROSENFELD, Albert. *Pro-longevity* New York: Avon, 1976.

WALFORD, Roy L. *Maximum Life Span* New York: W. W. Norton, 1983.
WOODRUFF, Diana S. *Can You Live To Be 100?* New York: Signet, 1977.

Part Six: The Ultra Face

COLGAN, Michael. *Your Personal Vitamin Profile* New York: Quill, 1982.
DEVINE, Elizabeth. *Appearances* London: Paitkus, 1982.
KASZAS, Joan. *Hair: Care For It and Keep It* New York: Barnes and Noble, 1973.
KLEIN, Arnold W., MD, Sternberg, James H., MD, and Bernstein, Paul. *The Skin Book*.
MAGNUS, I. A. *Dermatological Photobiology* Oxford: Blackwell Scientific Press, 1976.
MOOR, Kendall H., MD, and Thompson, Sally. *The Surgical Beauty Racket* Toronto: George J. McLeod, 1978.
PEARSON, Dirk, and Shaw, Sandy. *Life Extension – A Practical Scientific Approach* New York: Warner Books, 1982.
RINZLER, Carol Ann. *Cosmetics: What the Ads Don't Tell You* New York: Charter, 1977.
SCIENCE ACTION COALITION. *Consumer's Guides to Cosmetics* New York: Anchor Books, 1980.
SCOTT, Byron T. *How to Remodel Your Body* Matteson, Ill.: Greatlake Living Press, 1975.
SPERBER, Perry, MD. *Treatment of the Ageing Skin and Dermal Defects* Springfield, Ill.: Charles C. Thomas, 1965.
STERNBERG, James, MD, Sternberg, Thomas, MD, and Bernstein, Paul. *Great Skin at Any Age* New York: St Martin's Press, 1982.
THE EDITORS OF PREVENTION MAGAZINE. *The Natural Ways to a Healthy Skin* Emmaus, Pa: Rodale Press, 1972.
THE EDITORS OF PREVENTION MAGAZINE. *Vitamins for Better Health* Emmaus, Pa: Rodale Press, 1982.
WAGNER, Kurt J., MD, and Imber, Gerald, MD. *Beauty By Design* New York: McGraw-Hill, 1979.
ZIZMOR, Jonathan, MD, and Foreman, John. *Super Hair* New York: Berkeley Books, 1978.

Part Seven: The Body Beautiful

BAHR, Frank. *The Acupressure Health Book* London: Unwin Paperbacks, 1982.
BARLOW, Wilfred. *The Alexander Principle: How to Use Your Body* London: Arrow Books, 1975.
BENNET, William, MD, and Gurin, Joel. *The Dieter's Dilemma* New York: Basic Books, 1982.

BRANNIN, Marilyn. *Your Body in Mind* London: Souvenir, 1982.

HILL, Ann, ed. *A Visual Encyclopedia of Unconventional Medicine* London: New English Library, 1979.

FELDENKRAIS, Moshe. *Awareness Through Movement* London: Penguin, 1977.

FISHER, John. *Body Magic* London: Hodder and Stoughton, 1979.

HESSEL, Sidi. *The Articulate Body* New York: St Martin's Press, 1978.

HITTLEMAN, Richard. *Richard Hittleman's Introduction to Yoga* New York: Bantam, 1969.

KNEIPP, Sebastian. My *Water Cure* Wellingborough, Northants: Thorsons, 1979.

LAW, Donald. *Sauna For Health* London: Geoffrey Cave Associates Ltd, 1978.

MICHENER, Leslie, and Donaldson, Gerald. *The Exercise Book* London: Penguin, 1978.

NEWTON DUNNE, Esme. *The Bodywork Book* London: Willow Books, 1982.

NOBLE, Elizabeth. *Essential Exercises for the Childbearing Year* London: John Murray, 1978.

PEARCE, Joseph Chilton. *Magical Child* London: Paladin, 1977.

VALNET, Jean. *The Practice of Aromatherapy* Saffron Walden: C.W. Daniel Co., 1982.

Glossary

Abscisic acid A plant hormone associated with dormancy and leaf fall.

Acetylcholine A neurotransmitter.

Adrenaline A hormone produced by the inner part of the adrenal glands in mammals.

Alkaloid A name applied to a group of alkaline nitrogenous substances found in dicotyledonous plants, which have important physiological effects on the human body. Morphine, quinine, caffeine and atropine are well-known examples.

Amino acids Organic acids containing nitrogen which are the building blocks of protein.

Androgens Hormones secreted by the testes, or created synthetically, which control masculinity. Present in both sexes but predominant in males.

Apiol A gentle sedative with aspirin-like effects.

Autogenic training A type of relaxation therapy which is generated by the individual and which is entirely under his or her control.

Bioflavonoids A group of brightly-coloured substances widely distributed in plants. As human nutrients they contribute to the structure of blood vessel walls. They are always associated with vitamin C and enhance its actions.

Borneol An alcohol used in the manufacture of perfume and incense.

Carbodymethylcellulose An indigestible cellulose complex which is used as a bulk laxative and also as a slimming aid.

Catecholamines A class of neurotransmitters in the sympathetic nervous system, closely allied to adrenaline. They include dopamine and noradrenaline.

Chelating agents Organic compounds that can remove from circulation certain polyvalent metallic ions by binding them into their molecular structure. They are used to remove heavy metals from the body.

Cholesterol A crystalline substance of a fatty nature found in the brain, nerves, liver, blood and bile: it is not easily soluble and is a possible factor in hardening of the arteries. One type of gall stones is composed of cholesterol.

Choline A chemical found in animal tissues and also produced synthetically. It is the basic constituent of lecithin and is classified with the vitamin B complex. It is a precursor nutrient for acetylcholine in the brain. Richest sources are dairy products.

Collagen Fibre in the connective tissue which supports the body; it constitutes 30–40 per cent of the body's protein. Collagen is the elastic part of skin and once laid down is not renewed or replaced; old collagen is less elastic than young. Its decline is related to stiffness of joints and laxity of skin with increasing age.

Corticoid hormones A name for several groups of natural hormones produced by the cortex or outer layer of the adrenal gland, and for synthetic compounds with similar actions.

Cystine and cysteine Sulphur-containing amino acids. Cysteine stimulates the immune system.

Dinitrochlorobenzene (DTB) A substance used to determine cellular immunity.

DNA (deoxyribonucleic acid) The double-helix molecule in the nuclei of cells which contains genetic information.

Dopamine A neurotransmitter closely related to adrenaline which increases cardiac output and kidney blood flow, and plays an important role in emotions, body movement, sexual behaviour and immune system function.

Elastin A protein similar to collagen and which is the chief component of the elastic fibres of connective tissue.

Endocrine system System composed of organs (glands) which make and secrete substances (hormones) directly into the blood-stream; these have important influences on general metabolic processes. Examples of endocrine glands are pituitary, thyroid, thymus, adrenals, ovaries, testes, pancreas.

Endorphins A group of neurotransmitters with morphine-like action which are secreted by one particular region of the brain.

Enkephalins A group of substances similar in make-up and function to endorphins.

Enzymes Any of numerous complex proteins produced by living cells and which act as catalysts in specific biochemical reactions, e.g. yeast is a living cell which produces enzymes which change sugar into alcohol; ptyalin is an enzyme produced in the saliva which changes starch into sugar.

Essential fatty acids Organic acids, including linoleic, linolenic and arachaclonic acid, which occur naturally in fats, waxes and oils and are required by the body for health.

Essential oil Fine, light, almost etheric complex hydrocarbons taken from the leaves, stem, fruit or flowers of plants. Carries a plant's fragrance and often its healing properties.

Fenchone A substance which gives the characteristic bitter taste of fennel oil.

Ferredoxin An iron-containing protein found in some cells and bacteria.

Folic acid A vitamin of the vitamin B complex that is found especially in green leafy vegetables, liver and yeast. Lack of folic acid in the diet results in anaemia.

Gibberellins Plant growth hormones.

Glycogen Animal starch; the form in which carbohydrate is stored in the liver and muscles and released as energy needs demand.

Haematoporphyrin An iron-free decomposition product of haemoglobin.

High-density lipoproteins (HDL) High-density lipoproteins are thought to act as scavenger lipoproteins carrying a cholesterol from cells for re-utilization or degradation. (*See also* Low-density lipoproteins (LDL).)

Hormone A product of glandular activity in cells that produces a specific effect on the activity of cells elsewhere in the body; for example, adrenaline, produced by the adrenal glands in moments of sudden fear. Many hormones are now also produced synthetically.

Hyoscyamine Sleep-inducing drug obtained from deadly night-shade and henbane.

Iatrogenic ('Doctor-caused') A disease condition arising from medical intervention.

Indoles Compounds produced by intestinal decomposition of certain proteins.

Inositol A member of the vitamin B complex which, in combination with choline, can be used in the body to make lecithin.

Interferon A protein produced by cells as a defence against viruses. Vitamin C stimulates its production.

Lactucin A substance found in lettuce.

L-arganine An essential amino acid found in most proteins.

Lecithin A waxy substance, a phospholipid, found in plant and animal cells. Has emulsifying, wetting and anti-oxidant properties, and neutralizes excess fat in the diet.

L-glutamine and glutamic acid Amino acids found in most proteins which are important in the chemistry of the brain.

Linoleic acid An essential fatty acid found in vegetable seeds (e.g. linseed) which is essential for nutrition.

Lipid A broad class of fats and fat-like substances that ranks with carbohydrate and protein as basic categories of food substances.

Lipoproteins Compounds made up of lipid and protein, including carbohydrate protein. *See also* High-density lipoproteins; low-density lipoproteins

L-ornithine An amino acid obtained from L-arginine.

Low-density lipoproteins Fatty proteins in the blood whose presence is used to measure atherosclerotic risk of heart disease. A high HDL/LDL ratio is considered preferable; a low HDL/LDL ratio is considered an indication of high risk.

Lymphokines Factors produced by lymphocytes that affect other lymphocytes and macrophages.

Lysine An essential amino acid necessary for growth.

Macrophages Large white cells present in most parts of the body, especially the skin, which engulf and destroy debris and micro-organisms. They also play an important part in the maintenance and repair of tissue.

Melanin A brown-to-black pigment which is a factor in skin and hair colour. Suntan, freckles, and flat brown spots on the skin of elderly people are examples of melanin deposits.

Methionine An amino acid found in most proteins and essential to humans.

Mitochondria Threadlike or rod-like intracellular bodies in which the processes which release energy for cell life are mainly concentrated.

Mucin A polysaccharide or mixture of glycoproteins – the chief constituent of mucus.

Mucoid Resembling mucus.

Mucopolysaccharides The group of complex saccharides which comprise mucin.

Mucoproteins A series of amino acid compounds found in mucus.

Neurotransmitter A substance released from nerve endings to carry over the nerve impulse from one nerve to another, or from nerve to muscle or gland, especially for memory and the control of sensory and muscular output signals.

Noradrenaline (US: Norepinephreme) Substance produced in the cortex of the adrenal glands, in much smaller quantities than adrenaline.

Nucleic acids The long chain structures which provide the chemical basis of gene codes and their translation into cell processes.

Oestrogens Hormones produced by the ovary; they are responsible for the changes in the body during ovulation and for the development of female characteristics.

Pantothenic acid A constituent of the vitamin B complex.

Para-aminobenzoic acid (PABA) A constituent of the vitamin B complex.

Pelletierine A substance found in the root bark of the pomegranate tree.

Phenol Carbolic acid – a strong disinfectant.

Phenylalanine An amino acid found in most proteins and an essential nutrient for humans.

Phytohormone A plant hormone.

Pinene An aromatic used in many essential oils.

Polymer A large molecule of regular pattern, comprising many identical molecules joined end-to-end in the same way. The molecular equivalent of a crystal.

Polypeptide A compound made up of two or more amino acids.

Precursor Specific substance required for the manufacture of another substance within the body.

Procaine A synthetic substance similar to the alkaloid cocaine.

Prostaglandins A group of complex fatty acids which occur in minute amounts in virtually all body tissues and act as local tissue hormones or neurotransmitters. So named because early examples were found in the prostate gland.

Proteolytic enzymes Enzymes responsible for breaking down proteins into simpler substances.

Resorcin A mild antiseptic used in hair lotions and some skin treatments. Should not be used for long periods on open surfaces.

RNA (Ribonucleic acid) A complex substance found in the nuclei of all living cells which transfers genetic information from DNA for use in cell processes.

Saccharides A class of sweet-tasting carbohydrates, e.g. glucose, ribose and sucrose.

Salicylic acid A corrosive chemical related to aspirin.

Secretin A hormone produced in the duodenum which promotes secretion of pancreatic juices.

Serotonin An inhibitory neurotransmitter. The amino acid tryptophan, found in milk, cheese and bananas, is its precursor.

Sinigrin An alkaloid found in black mustard seed.

Thiamine Vitamin B1.

Thymosin Hormone secreted by the thyroid gland.

T-lymphocytes A variety of white blood cells which have been 'trained' in the thymus gland.

Triglycerides Combinations of glycerine with any three fatty acids.

Tryptamine A derivative of tryptophan.

Tryptophan An essential amino acid. (*See* Serotonin.)

Tyrosine An essential amino acid.

Vitamin An essential nitrogen-containing micronutrient, without which an enzyme reaction would not work. Distinct from amino acids which are macronutrients, actual building *materials*, whereas micronutrients are building *tools*.

Index

Abdominal Hold (exercise), 269–70
Abkhazians, the, 175–6
abscisic acid, 86, 297
acetaldehydes, 184, 186, 187
acetylcholine, 133, 141, 142, 143, 144, 204
acidophilus, 38, 39
acne, 28, 213, 217–19
acupressure, 257, 258
acupuncture face therapy, 246–7
additives, food, 17, 84, 99
adenosine triphosphate (ATP), 44, 47
adrenal gland, 127, 202
adrenaline, 51, 127, 133, 141, 142, 297
    excess, 49
advertisements, 12, 75
ageing (see also skin), 7, 173–4, 175
    attitudes to, 23–4, 155–6, 178
    diet and, 175–9, 181–2, 185–7, 191–2
    and exercise, 51–2, 179–82
    illness and, 10, 14, 146–7, 155, 174
    neurotransmitters and, 146–7, 148
    nutritional supplements and, 187–91
    rejuvenation techniques, 193–205
aggression: and catecholamines, 141–2
AHA (fruit acid) skin care, 191, 210
air pollution, 25, 28–30, 144
alcohol, 12, 13, 34–5, 130, 184, 187, 216
    dependence on, 116, 143, 148, 162
Alexander Technique, 159, 165–9, 252, 270
alfalfa, 88, see sprouts
algae, alginates, see seaweed
alkaloids, 297
allergies, 75, 77, 85
    and mental and emotional problems 113–14
    and overweight, 265
almonds, 146
    Almond Tonic (recipe), 94
alopecia, 233–4
aluminium poisoning, 29, 31, 114, 184, 187
    amino acids and, 147
amino acids, 102, 141, 143, 145, 146–9, 297
anacardic acid, anacardiol, 117
anaemia, 29, 31, 200, 226–7
Anderson, James, 50

androgens, 218, 297
androstenol, 262
angina, see heart disease
antacids, aluminium in, 29
antibiotics, 219
anti-depressants, see under depression
anti-oxidants, 185–6, 204–5
    anti-pollutant, 37–8
    and hair loss, 236–7
    for skin, 191–2, 216, 219–20
anxiety: food allergies and, 113, 114
    see depression; stress
apiol, 117, 120, 297
appetite suppressants, 146, 268
    exercise as, 46–7
apples, 18, 38, 266
    juice, 89
arsenic, 187
arteriosclerosis: caffeine and, 105
    cross-linking and, 183
    and diet, 100, 101, 103, 104
arthritis: cell therapy for, 200
    clay treatments for, 255
    cross-linking and, 27
    and diet, 85, 100, 119, 120
    and exercise, 58, 65
    and Gerovital-H3 therapy, 194, 195
Aslan, Anna, 193–4, 195, 196
Assiogioli, Roberto, 15
asthma, 58, 150, 162
Astrand, Per-Olaf, 56
AT, see autogenic training
atheromatous process, 51
ATP, see adenosine triphosphate
autogenic training (AT), 159–64
avocados, 94, 186
    Avocado Smoothie (soup), 96
Axelrod, Julius, 46

Bailey, Covert: Fit or Fat, 65
baldness, see hair, loss of